Overcoming Teenage Low Mood and Depression

ach

D1136247

2618142

Overcoming Teenage Low Mood and Depression

A Five Areas Approach

Dr Nicky Dummett MBBChir BA (Hons)
MRCPsych DCH MMedSc
Consultant Child and Adolescent
Psychiatrist,
Leeds Primary Care Trust, UK

Dr Chris Williams MBChB BSc MMEdSc MD
FRCPSYCH
Senior Lecturer and Honorary
Consultant Psychiatrist,
Section of Psychological Medicine,
University of Glasgow Medical School,
Glasgow, UK

Helping you to help yourself
www.livinglifetothefull.com
www.fiveareas.com

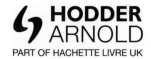
HODDER
ARNOLD
PART OF HACHETTE LIVRE UK

First published in Great Britain in 2008 by
Hodder Arnold, an imprint of Hodder Education
Part of Hachette Livre UK, 338 Euston Road, London NW1 3BH

http://www.hoddereducation.com

British Library Cataloguing in Publication Data
A catalogue record for this book is available from the British Library

Library of Congress Cataloging-in-Publication Data
A catalog record for this book is available from the Library of Congress

ISBN-13 978-0-340-94657-2

1 2 3 4 5 6 7 8 9 10

Commissioning Editor: Philip Shaw
Project Editor: Clare Patterson
Production Controller: Karen Tate
Cover Design: Amina Dudhia

Typeset in 11pt Frutiger by Pantek Arts Ltd., Maidstone, Kent.
Printed and bound in Malta.

What do you think about this book? Or any other Hodder Arnold title?

Please visit our website: **www.hoddereducation.com** or send comments to feedback@fiveareas.com

New ways of accessing the workbooks

Other linked resources are available from **www.fiveareas.com**

Buying the books in bulk: Bulk copies of the book are available at discounted rates direct from the publisher.
5–30 copies: 25%
31–50 copies: 30%
51–100 copies: 40%
100–200 copies: 45%
200+ copies: 50%

To take advantage of these reduced rates please contact:
Jane MacRae, Sales Development Manager, Hodder Headline, 338 Euston Road, London NW1 3BH. Tel: +44 (0) 20 7873 6146; e-mail: **jane.macrae@hodder.co.uk**

Details of other ways of delivering the course are available at **www.livinglifetothefull.com** are **www.fiveareas.com**

Contents

Foreword

Young people often feel down, sad or unhappy for short periods of time, although for some this unfortunately becomes a way of life. Feelings of unhappiness persist, become intense and start to interfere with everyday activities. Low mood and depression take over, with school work, social life, friendships and family relationships all being affected.

Many of these young people would benefit from some form of help but undoubtedly are often deterred from seeking help by the stigma associated with mental health problems. There is also poor recognition and understanding of adolescent depression within general practice and by community professionals. It is therefore not surprising that comparatively few young people are referred and seen for treatment by specialist child mental health services. This highlights the need to increase the availability of good, user-friendly, theoretically based materials which can be more directly accessed and used by young people.

Overcoming Teenage Low Mood and Depression: A Five Areas Approach is a welcome and much needed self-help manual designed for young people with depression and low mood. It is based on the very successful self-help format used in *Overcoming Depression and Low Mood* but has been specifically adapted and written for use with young people. The material is based on the theoretical model of cognitive behaviour therapy (CBT), which has been identified as being effective in mild and moderate depression by the National Institute of Health and Clinical Excellence (NICE 2005).[1] *Overcoming Teenage Low Mood and Depression* uses a 'five areas' approach to help young people understand how they are feeling. They are helped to discover the relationship between people and the events that happen, what they think about these, how these thoughts make them feel, the physical symptoms these produce and the effect of these on their behaviour. Developing this understanding is an important first step that can help a young person to make sense of how they are feeling. This understanding can in itself be very empowering and can help the young person realise that they can make changes that will help them to feel better.

Through a series of attractive workbooks *Overcoming Teenage Low Mood and Depression* provides the young person with opportunities to explore some of the important areas that contribute to the development and maintenance of low mood and to develop skills that will help them to feel better. There are workbooks to help understand the importance of activity; to identify, challenge and modify extreme and unhelpful thinking; to develop helpful problem-solving skills; and to understand how to build supportive relationships and how to manage some of the physiological symptoms associated with low mood, such as disturbed or disrupted sleep. There is also a helpful workbook for families and friends that provides useful information about depression and low mood, and many practical ideas about what they can do to help.

Overcoming Teenage Low Mood and Depression is written specifically for young people and provides a wealth of useful information, helpful self-assessment tasks, and many practical ideas and activities. This practical emphasis is very engaging and helps the

[1] NICE (2005) *Depression in Children and Young People: Identification and Management in Primary, Community and Secondary Care*. National Clinical Practice no. 28. London: NICE.

young person to explore each theme in a logical and structured way. The workbooks can be tailored to the particular needs of the young person who decides which areas are important and the order in which they wish to approach them. *Overcoming Teenage Low Mood and Depression* also offers considerable flexibility and can be used independently by young people on their own or as part of an intervention facilitated by a primary care or mental health professional.

This flexible and user-friendly book is an excellent resource for young people and professionals. I am sure that *Overcoming Teenage Low Mood and Depression* will help many young people learn skills that will help them to overcome their low mood and depression.

Paul Stallard
Professor of Child and Family Mental Health
University of Bath

Introduction

Welcome to *Overcoming Teenage Low Mood and Depression: A Five Areas Approach*. This book is based on many years' experience of work using this approach. It uses a self-help approach that many young people prefer as it allows them to lead their own recovery, with support from other key people. These people might include trusted friends or relatives, and school, youth or healthcare workers.

The book uses a wide range of ways to help support readers to help themselves. It does this by providing clearly described practical tools to help them make changes. The hope is that you will find encouragement and feel empowered to make changes yourself.

Who is this book for?

The book can be used by many different people. You may be someone using the resources for yourself, or perhaps you are a close friend or family member wanting to know more about low mood and depression. Many healthcare workers also use workbooks in this series to support those they work with. Our experience has shown that these books can be used by people with problems ranging from mild distress through to more severe depression. The treatment approach involves **reading** the course workbooks and also **working** on problems. If your concentration, energy or motivation levels are far lower than usual and you find it very hard to keep your mind on things or to make changes, then it may not be the right time to use this course. If you find that you're struggling to use the workbooks, or you feel worse as you work through, them please discuss this with your own doctor or other healthcare worker. The workbooks are not meant to replace getting the right level of support for more severe mental health problems.

How does the book work?

Have you ever had the experience of someone you know saying 'What you said last time really made a great difference', yet you can't remember quite what you said? Perhaps something similar has happened to you when you have been mulling over a problem and a friend or relative has said something that really helped put things into perspective? This common experience indicates that providing the right information or question can make a real difference to how we feel. The concept of using sequences of effective questions and information is the basis of cognitive behaviour therapy (CBT; a kind of talking treatment), which has proven effectiveness in the treatment of depression.

What will you learn?

Overcoming Teenage Low Mood and Depression: A Five Areas Approach contains workbooks that address all the main problem areas affected during times of low mood. The workbooks will help you discover why you feel as you do, and also teach you key skills that you can use to improve things.

You will:

- Discover why you feel as you do
- Learn how to boost your motivation to change
- Learn how to become more active and rediscover the fun in life
- Learn how to build exercise into your life to combat low mood
- Learn how to develop helpful responses to life stresses
- Discover how unhelpful activities can drag you down
- Restart doing things you've been avoiding
- Develop better problem-solving skills
- Learn how to change negative and undermining thinking
- Learn how to rebalance relationships by becoming more assertive
- Learn how to build and rebuild relationships
- Discover how to sleep better
- Find out more about alcohol and street drugs and how they affect people
- Understand the role of anti-depressant medication
- Learn how to plan for the future in order to stay well.

The last workbook is aimed at friends and relatives and it describes how to best offer support.

There is no right or wrong way to use the workbooks. Many people find it most helpful to read the first two workbooks in Section 1 (*Understanding why I feel as I do* and *Why bother changing?*) to help gain an overview of the approach. This will also help you to decide which of the Making Changes workbooks in Part 2 of the book you should read. You can use as many or as few workbooks in the course as you wish. A key to creating change in your life is **using** the workbooks and **putting what you learn into practice**.

A word of encouragement

No-one is immune to depression. Low mood and depression are common and affect many people. They can affect each of us in all sorts of ways. Fortunately it has now become clear that changing certain thoughts and behaviour patterns can have a significant effect on improving how we feel. The content of this guide is based on the CBT approach. This has identified effective ways of tackling many of the common symptoms and problems faced when we feel low. Don't worry though about this complex language – we have made sure that the workbooks are written in a way that you can understand. Each workbook will teach you invaluable information about how low mood and depression affect you. They also will help you learn some practical skills that you can use to bring about positive change. The workbooks aim to help you to **regain a sense of control** over how you feel.

However, sometimes making changes is easier said (or written) than done. All of us feel discouraged and overwhelmed from time to time. This is even more likely to occur in times of low mood. We want to encourage you to try to make a commitment to use this course and to keep at it even if you feel discouraged or stuck for a time. To do this you will need to **pace yourself** by using a step-by-step approach. Bear in mind what your motivation and energy levels allow you to do so you don't bite off more than you can chew. This will help you to get as much from the course as you can at the moment.

The *Why bother changing?* workbook gives some suggestions of how you can **pace things**, and also some suggestions of what you can do if you're struggling.

New on-line resources

 A new on-line free resource has been written to support users of the course. This is available at the Living Life to the Full website (**www.livinglifetothefull.com**). Also, a range of linked resources are available from **www.fiveareas.com**.

A note about copyright

The materials once purchased in book form may be copied by the user as many times as required for use by themselves, or (if a practitioner) in clinical practice or in training.

Acknowledgements

No sets of materials such as these could have been written by just two people. The creation of this course has developed out of work in teaching and working with young people, and also extensive work using self-help in adults. They would not have been possible without the support, feedback and stimulation we have received from a variety of colleagues over the years. We also owe an immense debt to the comments and feedback of people using these materials themselves as well as colleagues who have attended various training workshops and asked difficult questions that have helped 'test' and improve the approach. We would also particularly like to thank Dr Paul Farrand, Steve Yelland, Phil Munroe and Keith Hibbert who have helpfully commented on previous versions of the workbooks.

The illustrations in the workbooks have been produced by Keith Chan (kchan75@hotmail.com). Thanks too to the staff at Hodder Headline who have supported the development of the series of new Five Areas materials which are being released over the next few years.

Finally, we wish to thank Paul, Sam, Sophie, Ben and Beverley, and Alison, Hannah and Andrew who have supported us during the writing of this book.

Dr Nicky Dummett and Dr Chris Williams
February 2008

PART 1

Understanding why I feel as I do

PART 1

Understanding
why I feel
as I do

Overcoming Teenage Low Mood and Depression

A Five Areas Approach

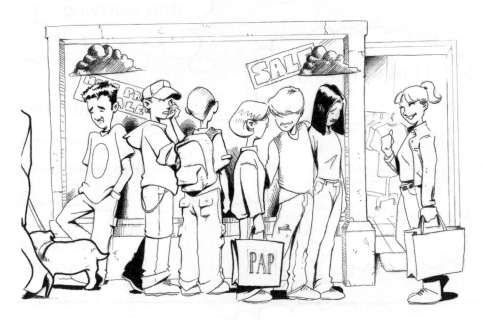

Understanding why I feel as I do

Helping you to help yourself
www.livinglifetothefull.com
www.fiveareas.com

Dr Nicky Dummett and Dr Chris Williams

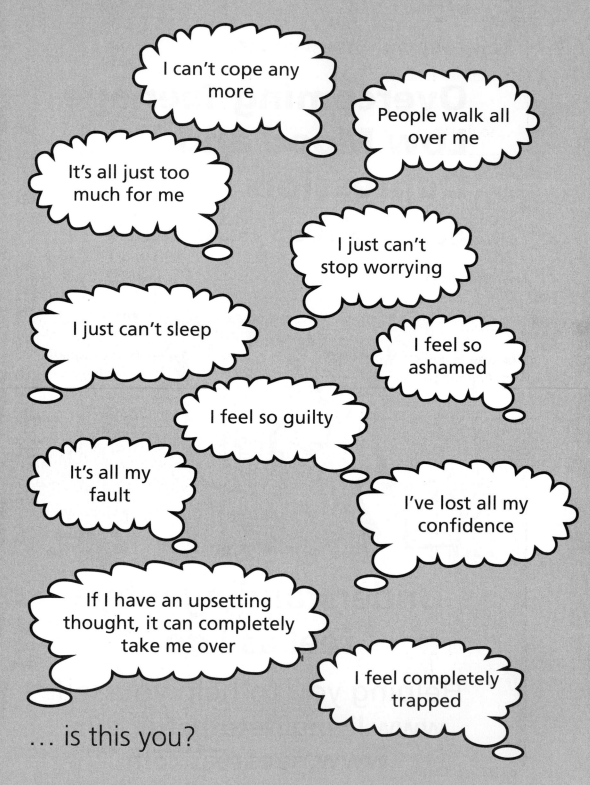

… is this you?

If it is … this **course is for you**.

This course will help you to:

- Find out about the causes of your low mood and stress

- Change the problem areas of your life

... so that you begin to feel better!

 How do I do this?

Use this course to plan **a step-by-step approach to recovery**.

Let's first look at how your problems have developed and where you are now.

How did things get to be like this?

One way of finding out how your problems have developed is to use a **time line**. An example is shown below.

 Example: Mark's time line

January: Everything was reasonably OK.

February: Increasing pressure of school work with exams coming up.

April: Bullying at school.

June: Struggling to cope, can't sleep; lying awake worrying about things. My GP suggests referral to a child and adolescent mental health service.

July: Told by them I have a depressive disorder.

Today: **Using the course – I want to make some changes**.

Task

Now it's your turn to have a go. Fill in your own time line below.

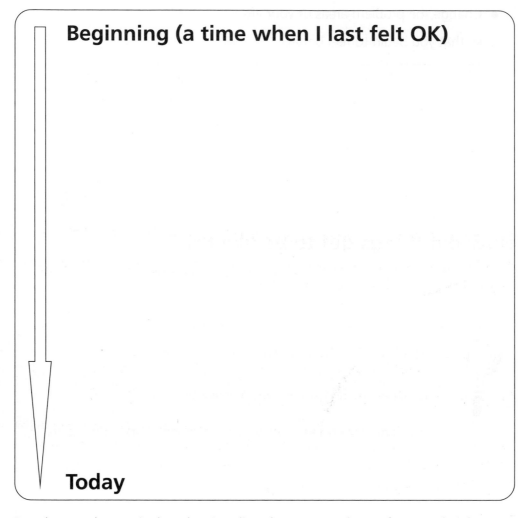

Beginning (a time when I last felt OK)

Today

But the good news is that the time line doesn't stop here. If you make changes from now on, things can be different.

Remember that anyone can have low mood or depression if their emotional balance gets upset.

 Has this happened to you?

Normally, we feel **able to cope** with the problems we face because we feel in balance. But when you feel low and distressed your balance is upset. Your problems can seem larger than they are, and you think you can't cope.

Out of balance – things feel worse and worse

In other words …

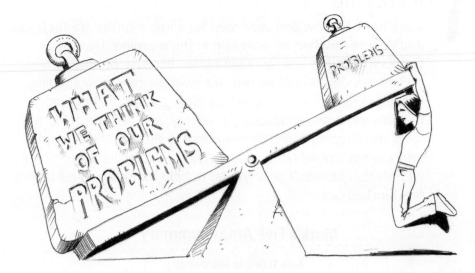

It's not just the situation or problem on its own that causes us to feel down or stressed. Instead it's **how we think about things** that makes us feel like we do.

Q Do I feel in balance at the moment?

Yes ☐   No ☐   Sometimes ☐

Using the Five Areas Approach

One helpful way of understanding how low mood and depression affect us is to think of the ways that they can affect different areas of our life. The **Five Areas** approach helps us to do this by examining in detail five important aspects of our life.

The five areas are:

- Area 1: **People and events** around us

- Area 2: Altered **thinking**

- Area 3: Altered **feelings** (also called moods or emotions)

- Area 4: Altered **physical symptoms** in our body

- Area 5: Altered **behaviour** or activity levels. This includes both the helpful things we do that make us feel better and the unhelpful things we do that backfire on how we feel.

Example: How low mood and depression affect Mark's life

Mark has been low and depressed for some months. He **feels** low and near tears when he wakes up in the morning. He often **thinks** that things will never get better. Because of how he feels he has changed his **behaviour**, for example he is now keeping himself to himself and is no longer playing football. **Physically** he's slowing down and lacking in energy, and he's picking at his food and sleeping badly. His behaviour is also affecting **people and events** around him, particularly his relationships. His mother worries that he won't do anything to help himself, and his friends feel blocked out.

Mark's Five Areas summary

Area 1: People and events
Arguments with my mother
Blocking out my friends

Area 2: Altered thinking
Things will never get better

Area 4: Altered physical symptoms
Slowed down and lacking energy
Gone off food
Sleeping really badly

Area 3: Altered feelings
Low and depressed
Near tears

Area 5: Altered behaviour
Keeping myself to myself
No longer playing football

Now try it out yourself. Can the Five Areas Approach help you understand the effect of low mood?

You can test whether this approach can help you work out the answer to 'Why do I feel as I do?'. Let's have a look at what's happening for you in each of the five areas in turn, starting with Area 1.

Area 1: People and events around us

All of us from time to time have problems with:

- Family and home
- Friends and other relationships
- School or college.

We also face practical problems such as dealing with other things that have happened in our life or with other people.

All these problems affect how we think, feel and behave.

 What's gone on for you in Area 1: People and events?

Family and home: Does this cause problems for me?

1   I find it hard to get on with one or more of my parents or carers.
     Often ☐   Sometimes ☐   No ☐

2   I find it hard to get on with another person or people in my family.
     Often ☐   Sometimes ☐   No ☐

3   Other people in my family don't get on.
     Often ☐   Sometimes ☐   No ☐

4   One or both of my parents or carers has been absent, left home or gone away.
     Often ☐   Sometimes ☐   No ☐

5   I am now living separately from some or all of my family.
     Often ☐   Sometimes ☐   No ☐

6   My family has housing problems (for example too small, may have to leave).
     Often ☐   Sometimes ☐   No ☐

7   My family has unemployment (joblessness) or money worries.
     Often ☐   Sometimes ☐   No ☐

8   I am (or we are) having problems with neighbours.
     Often ☐   Sometimes ☐   No ☐

Friends and other relationships

9   I've fallen out with one or more of my friends.
     Often ☐   Sometimes ☐   No ☐

10 There is no-one around whom I can really talk to.

Often ☐   Sometimes ☐   No ☐

11 A person or people important to me has been out of contact or gone away.

Often ☐   Sometimes ☐   No ☐

Practical problems

12 I or someone else close to me has physical or mental health problems.

Often ☐   Sometimes ☐   No ☐

13 I or someone else close to me has drug or alcohol problems.

Often ☐   Sometimes ☐   No ☐

14 I (or we) face other practical problems at the moment.

Often ☐   Sometimes ☐   No ☐

School or college

15 I have problems with school or college work, exams or tests.

Often ☐   Sometimes ☐   No ☐

16 I find it hard to attend or stay in school or college.

Often ☐   Sometimes ☐   No ☐

17 I have recently changed school or college.

Often ☐   Sometimes ☐   No ☐

18 I have problems with other people my age at school or college.

Often ☐   Sometimes ☐   No ☐

19 I have problems with staff at my school or college.

Often ☐   Sometimes ☐   No ☐

20 I'm being bullied or picked on.

Often ☐   Sometimes ☐   No ☐

Things that have happened in my life: Are any still happening?

21 Someone has been doing or saying things they shouldn't so that I didn't or don't feel safe.

Often ☐   Sometimes ☐   No ☐

22 Something else has happened that has really upset or harmed me or someone close to me.

Often ☐   Sometimes ☐   No ☐

Task

Now write here about any other problems you may have. Also, write in more detail about any of your answers. Give the question number and when the problem happened. Is it still happening?

Use an extra sheet of paper if you need to or use the 'My notes' pages at the back of this workbook.

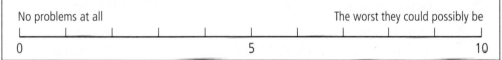

Summary of my people and events review

Having answered these questions, overall, do I have (or have I had) problems in Area 1: People and events? For example, if you found that you have many problems in this area you might rate yourself 8 or 9. If you have very few problems in this area you might rate yourself only 1 or 2.

No problems at all   The worst they could possibly be

0   5   10

What next for problems in Area 1?

You or your family and friends may find reading the *Ideas for families and friends* workbook helpful in getting you thinking. If this is an area you wish to work on, workbooks in the course will help you to rebalance relationships (the *Being assertive* and *Building relationships* workbooks) and to begin tackling practical problems (*Practical problem solving* workbook).

Do I need extra help from other people?

Sometimes, we can't sort all of our problems with people and events ourselves. We may need other people to change too – or we may even need to look for help from outside. For example, if you or someone close to you is at risk of immediate, significant harm (such as abuse or serious self-harm), then you may need others to help you.

If you are worried or concerned, **it's better to ask for help or advice than do nothing**. Try to think of an adult you trust and you can talk to straight away. Your general practitioner (GP) or social services or even your local emergency department can be helpful. There will be office hours and 24-hour emergency telephone numbers for these locally. There are also 24-hour help-lines that you can call just to talk things over without the number appearing on the phone bill (for example ChildLine and the National Society for the Prevention of Cruelty to Children (NSPCC) Child Protection Helpline). Contact details for sources of help are given at the end of this workbook (pages **27–30**).

Area 2: Altered thinking

When we are feeling down, how we **think** changes. We tend to lose confidence and find it more difficult to make decisions. We may keep mulling over things we have and haven't done. We can end up viewing everything in a negative and unhelpful way. Our thinking becomes:

- Extreme
- Unhelpful.

Example: How you think can affect your behaviour

Imagine that someone you are talking to looks vacant for a moment. You might think 'They find me boring'. And so you start to feel low and anxious and your body feels tensed up. You might then change your behaviour by avoiding eye contact and answering questions with short replies. You might try to break off the conversation and leave. If, however, you thought 'They look really tired', you would feel and behave differently.

We may also spend too much time **dwelling** on our worries, turning them over in our mind again and again. Remember that people rarely come up with good solutions while doing this because it makes us feel much worse. And our thinking just gets more negative.

My unhelpful thinking patterns

 Have you noticed any of these common unhelpful patterns of thinking in your life?

Unhelpful thinking pattern	Do I ever think this way? (Tick box if yes and write down an example)
Bias against myself For example, being very self-critical; overlooking my strengths; seeing myself as not coping; not recognising my achievements	☐
Putting a negative slant on things (negative mental filter) For example, seeing things through dark tinted glasses; seeing the glass as being half empty rather than half full; that whatever I've done in the week it's never enough to give me a sense of achievement; tending to focus on the bad side of everyday situations	☐
Having a gloomy view of the future For example, thinking that things will stay bad or get even worse; tending to feel that things will go wrong; always looking for the next thing to fail	☐
Jumping to the worst conclusion (catastrophic thinking) For example, tending to feel that the very worst will happen; often thinking that I will fail really badly	☐
Having a negative view about how others see me (mind-reading) For example, often thinking that others don't like me, or think badly of me for no particular reason	☐

Unhelpful thinking pattern	Do I ever think this way? (Tick box if yes and write down an example)
Unfairly taking responsibility for things For example, thinking I should take the blame if things go wrong; feeling guilty about things that are not really my fault; thinking I'm responsible for everyone else	☐
Making extreme statements/rules For example: ● Using the words 'always' and 'never' a lot to summarise things ● If a bad thing happens, saying 'Just typical' because it seems this always happens ● Making myself a lot of 'must', 'should' 'ought' or 'got to' rules ● Believing I must always push myself to do things well	☐

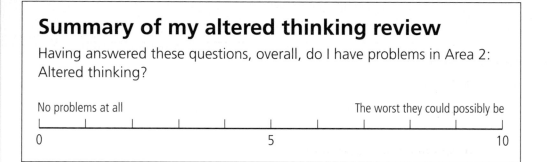

Summary of my altered thinking review

Having answered these questions, overall, do I have problems in Area 2: Altered thinking?

No problems at all   The worst they could possibly be

0   5   10

What next?

If this is an area you wish to work on, the *Noticing and changing extreme and unhelpful thinking workbook* will help you to identify and change these ways of thinking.

Area 3: Altered feelings

Our feelings or **emotions** can be very strong (and hard to bear at times). This is a chance for you to think about how you have been feeling. The good news is that by making changes to other areas, you can improve how you feel. If you measure how you feel now and then after you've worked through some of this course, you will be able to see which things have made a positive difference.

Q What emotional changes have you noticed over the past two weeks?

- Lowness or sadness

  Yes ☐   No ☐   Sometimes ☐

- Lack of enjoyment or pleasure in things

  Yes ☐   No ☐   Sometimes ☐

- Loss of all feelings, for example noticing no feelings at all

  Yes ☐   No ☐   Sometimes ☐

- Guilt

  Yes ☐   No ☐   Sometimes ☐

- Worry, stress, tension, anxiety or panic

  Yes ☐   No ☐   Sometimes ☐

- Anger or irritability with yourself or others

  Yes ☐   No ☐   Sometimes ☐

- Shame or embarrassment

  Yes ☐   No ☐   Sometimes ☐

- Other (write down here):

Summary of my altered feelings review

Having answered these questions, overall, do I have problems in Area 3: Altered feelings?

No problems at all   The worst they could possibly be

0   5   10

Area 4: Altered physical symptoms

Usually, when people feel very low emotionally, they also complain about physical symptoms (or other upset, for example anxiety).

Q Which physical symptoms have you noticed over the past two weeks?

- Wakening earlier than usual

  Yes ☐   No ☐   Sometimes ☐

- Finding it hard to go to sleep

  Yes ☐   No ☐   Sometimes ☐

- Waking up in the night

  Yes ☐   No ☐   Sometimes ☐

- An unusually increased or decreased appetite

  Yes ☐   No ☐   Sometimes ☐

- Increased or decreased weight

  Yes ☐   No ☐   Sometimes ☐

- Reduced energy

  Yes ☐   No ☐   Sometimes ☐

- Constipation

  Yes ☐   No ☐   Sometimes ☐

- Poor concentration

  Yes ☐   No ☐   Sometimes ☐

- Physical agitation

  Yes ☐   No ☐   Sometimes ☐

- Reduced enjoyment of things

  Yes ☐   No ☐   Sometimes ☐

- Other (write down here):

Summary of my physical symptoms review

Having answered these questions, overall, do I have problems in Area 4: Altered physical symptoms?

No problems at all   The worst they could possibly be

|—|—|—|—|—|—|—|—|—|—|

0   5   10

The good news is that by making changes in other areas, we can improve how we feel physically. If you measure your physical symptoms now and after you have worked through some of the rest of this course, you will be able to see which things have made a positive difference. You can also find some advice about how to tackle problems with sleeping in the *Overcoming sleep problems* workbook.

Area 5: Altered behaviour

You have already worked hard thinking about the first four of the five areas in your Five Areas assessment – well done! This section deals with the final area of your Five Areas assessment – altered behaviour (things that we do).

Some things that we do can make matters worse, but there are things we do that can help us feel better. The ways in which your altered behaviour may worsen your low mood or depression are:

- **Reducing your activity** (not doing much)
- **Avoiding** (or **escaping** from) doing things that seem too difficult
- Not doing the helpful things you do
- Starting to do **unhelpful things** (for example isolating yourself, shouting at people or even using alcohol or street drugs to block how you feel).

All these unhelpful changes in our behaviour can worsen how we feel.

Key point

Making changes in your behaviour and activity levels are usually some of the most helpful things you can do to boost how you feel.

First type of altered behaviour: Reduced activity

When we feel down, it's hard to do things because of:

- Low energy and tiredness
- Little sense of enjoyment or achievement even when we do manage to do things
- Negative thinking about things ('I just can't be bothered', 'What's the point'?).

This leads to **reduced activity,** which means we reduce or stop doing everyday life activities – things that normally make us feel better by bringing us a sense of fun, enjoyment or **pleasure**, a sense of **achievement** or a feeling of **closeness** to other people ... and so we feel worse and worse.

My reduced activities

Q Have I cut down or stopped **everyday life activities** that most people my age would normally be doing (for example washing, dressing, eating properly, sleeping regularly, having hobbies, relaxing, doing homework and tasks I have to do, getting out and about, going to school or college, socialising with family or friends)?

Yes ☐   No ☐   Sometimes ☐

Q Have I reduced or stopped doing things that previously gave me a sense of **pleasure**?

Yes ☐   No ☐   Sometimes ☐

Q Have I reduced or stopped doing things that previously gave me a sense of **achievement**?

Yes ☐   No ☐   Sometimes ☐

Q Have I reduced or stopped doing things that previously gave me a sense of **closeness** to others?

Yes ☐   No ☐   Sometimes ☐

Q Overall, has this worsened how I feel?

Yes ☐   No ☐   Sometimes ☐

Write down any examples here:

The good news is that once you've noticed that this is true for you, you can start working on tackling reduced activity in a planned, step-by-step way. You will find out how to do this in the workbook *Doing things that make me feel good*.

Second type of altered behaviour: Avoiding or escaping from things

We often start to **avoid** or **escape** from people, places and situations that worry us. But this teaches us the unhelpful rule that the **only** way of dealing with a difficult situation is to avoid it or escape from it. So it becomes even harder to face similar problems next time round. We also don't get to find out that our worst fears don't happen. So, avoidance and escaping make us feel worse and also undermine our confidence.

Avoiding or escaping from people, places or situations

Q Am I avoiding people or avoiding doing certain things?

Yes ☐   No ☐   Sometimes ☐

Q Has this reduced my confidence in things?

Yes ☐   No ☐   Sometimes ☐

Q Has my life become increasingly restricted?

Yes ☐   No ☐   Sometimes ☐

Q Am I avoiding conversations I need to have?

Yes ☐   No ☐   Sometimes ☐

Q Overall has this worsened how I feel?

Yes ☐   No ☐   Sometimes ☐

Write down any examples here:

The good news is that if you have noticed this is true for you, you can start working on tackling avoidance and escaping in a planned, step-by-step way. You will find out how to do this in the workbook *Restarting things we've avoided*.

Third type of altered behaviour: Dropping helpful things we do

Helpful behaviours include things such as:

- Talking to friends or family for support and yet also being firm about when you need to sort things out yourself without other people taking over

- Recognising times when you have been too hard on yourself

- Still doing activities that give pleasure or a sense of achievement or closeness to other people, such as doing things you enjoy and meeting friends

- Checking the internet for sensible information or reading or using self-help materials to find out more about the causes and ways to help low mood and depression

- Going to see a doctor or other healthcare practitioner to discuss whether you may need extra help

- If you have a personal spiritual faith, perhaps praying or asking others to pray for you, reading your scriptures, and focusing on verses that confirm love and support from God.

My helpful behaviours

Q Have I dropped any helpful behaviours?

Yes ☐   No ☐   Sometimes ☐

Write down any examples here:

Q Is this worsening how I feel?

Yes ☐   No ☐   Sometimes ☐

Write down any examples here:

Am I still doing any helpful behaviours?

Q Am I still doing anything that improves how I feel?

Yes ☐   No ☐   Sometimes ☐

Q Overall has this improved how I feel?

Yes ☐   No ☐   Sometimes ☐

Write down any examples here:

If you've answered 'Yes' or 'Sometimes' to the questions above, you are still responding in helpful ways. Well done! You can try to build even more of these helpful responses back into your life to help yourself feel better. You can find out more about ways of building helpful behaviours in the workbooks called *Helpful things we do* and *Doing things that make me feel good*.

Fourth type of altered behaviour: Unhelpful things we do

Sometimes we may do things that make us feel better at first but in the longer term backfire and make us feel worse. Do you think you do any of the following **unhelpful behaviours**?

- Withdrawing into yourself and cutting yourself off from your friends or family

- Neglecting yourself (for example by not washing or eating properly)

- Finding yourself tempted to do things that you know are unwise or wrong (for example deliberately taking risks, picking fights or going behind people's backs)

- Acting out of frustration or anger to harm or hurt others; that is, acting in ways to test out the love or support of others (for example being rude and critical, or pushing people away to see how much they really want to support you)

- Using alcohol or street drugs to block how you feel

- Harming yourself as a way of blocking how you feel (for example self-cutting).

My unhelpful behaviours

Q Am I doing some things to try to make me feel better immediately?

Yes ☐   No ☐   Sometimes ☐

Q Are some of these things unhelpful later on?

Yes ☐   No ☐   Sometimes ☐

Q Overall have unhelpful behaviours worsened how I feel?

Yes ☐   No ☐   Sometimes ☐

Write down any examples here:

If you have answered 'Yes' or 'Sometimes' to all the questions above, you are experiencing a **vicious circle** of unhelpful behaviour. A key thing to watch out for is how we all tend to get into a habit of reacting to difficult situations in certain ways. By watching out for any **unhelpful behaviours** that we keep falling into and by choosing to respond differently we can make large changes in how we feel. You will find out more about reducing unhelpful behaviours in the workbook *Unhelpful things we do*.

Now think of all the altered behaviours you have thought about until now together.

Summary of my behaviours review

Having answered the all the questions, overall, do I have problems in Area 5: Altered behaviours?

No problems at all   The worst they could possibly be

0   5   10

Let's look at the whole picture again

Think again of your review of all of the **five areas** and how you have rated yourself in each.

Q Overall, do I have (or have I had) problems in Area 1: People and events?

No problems at all   The worst they could possibly be

0   5   10

Q Overall, do I have problems in Area 2: Altered thinking?

No problems at all   The worst they could possibly be

0   5   10

Q Overall, do I have problems in Area 3: Altered feelings?

No problems at all   The worst they could possibly be

0   5   10

Q Overall, do I have problems in Area 4: Altered physical symptoms?

No problems at all   The worst they could possibly be

0   5   10

Q Overall, do I have problems in Area 5: Altered behaviours?

No problems at all   The worst they could possibly be

0   5   10

 What have I learnt from this review?

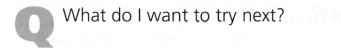

Q What do I want to try next?

What next?

Remember that the **Five Areas assessment** isn't intended to make you feel worse. Rather, by helping you think of how you are now, this assessment can help you plan the areas you need to focus on to bring about change. The good news is that all these areas are linked and so changing any one of them will bring about change in others. So if you aim to **alter any of these areas**, it will help lift your low mood and help you tackle feeling low or stressed.

In the figure below write in the boxes one or two words to remind you of the most important changes you've noticed in yourself in each area and the overall size of your problem (out of 10) for each area.

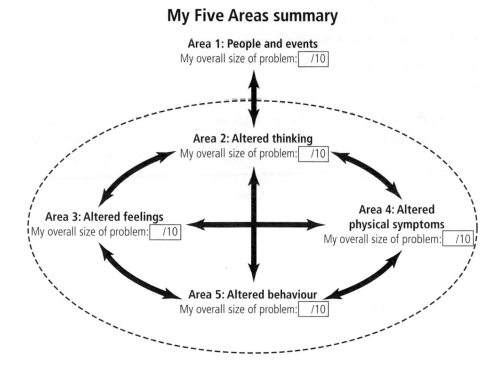

My Five Areas summary

Area 1: People and events
My overall size of problem: ☐ /10

Area 2: Altered thinking
My overall size of problem: ☐ /10

Area 3: Altered feelings
My overall size of problem: ☐ /10

Area 4: Altered physical symptoms
My overall size of problem: ☐ /10

Area 5: Altered behaviour
My overall size of problem: ☐ /10

So where do I start?

The workbooks in this course can help you begin to tackle each of the five problem areas of depression. A key to success is **not to try tackling everything at once**. Slow steady steps are more likely to result in improvement than being too enthusiastic at the start and then running out of steam. So try to tackle things one thing at a time by setting yourself:

● Short-term targets: changes you can make today, tomorrow and next week

● Medium-term targets: changes to be put in place over the next few weeks

● Long-term targets: where you want to be in six months or a year.

Which workbook should I try first?

Use your Five Areas assessment **to help you decide** which workbook to try first. Pick just one area and one workbook of the course first. This also means that you are actively at first choosing **not** to focus on other areas.

We recommend that people **first focus on**:

● **Changing behaviours** (*Doing things that make me feel good*, *Using exercise to boost how I feel*, *Helpful things we do* and *Unhelpful things we do* workbooks)

● **Building up useful skills** (*Practical problem solving* and *Being assertive* workbooks)

Then try to change negative thinking (*Noticing and changing extreme and unhelpful thinking* workbook). Focusing too early on negative thoughts can make you feel worse. If you have a close family member or friend you'd like to help you in using the course, ask them to read the *Ideas for families and friends* workbook; you may also find it helpful yourself.

Workbook	Plan to read	Tick when completed
Understanding why I feel as I do	☐	☐
Why bother changing?	☐	☐
Doing things that make me feel good	☐	☐
Using exercise to boost how I feel	☐	☐
Helpful things we do	☐	☐
Unhelpful things we do	☐	☐
Restarting things we've avoided	☐	☐
Practical problem solving	☐	☐
Noticing and changing extreme and unhelpful thinking	☐	☐
Being assertive	☐	☐
Building relationships	☐	☐
Overcoming sleep problems	☐	☐
Alcohol, drugs and me	☐	☐
Understanding and using anti-depressant medication	☐	☐
Planning for the future	☐	☐
Ideas for families and friends: how can I offer the best support?	☐	☐

Key point

Repeat your Five Areas assessment after using each workbook **to help you decide where to go next**.

How do I know whether I need extra help?

We recommend that if you're using these workbooks, ideally you have someone to support you in doing it. If you have somebody supporting you, discuss what you have been doing with them. If things seem to be worsening or you feel stuck then you may need extra help.

Extra help is especially important for:

- **Severe depression**, for example continuing low mood, tearfulness, not eating or drinking much at all or a big loss of weight despite attempts to improve things

- Strong urges to **self-harm** or feeling really **hopeless or suicidal** about the future

- Other **dangerous behaviours**, for example risk taking or threats of harm to others

- A possibility of immediate or longer-term significant harm or injury to a child or young person by someone else; that is, **physical, emotional or sexual abuse or neglect**

- **Severe withdrawal from life activities**, for example a lot of absences from school.

There are also other situations where extra help might be needed. If either you or the person supporting you is still worried that something else needs to be done, then it's important to ask for help at least in deciding whether more help is needed.

It is better to ask for help or advice than do nothing.

Getting extra help

You can ask:

- **Someone you can trust**. Try to think of an adult you trust to talk to. You may find it's easier to talk to someone **outside** your closest friends and family. Don't feel guilty if you feel like this, because it's normal – many people feel the same way.

- **Your family doctor or GP**. Your GP can offer medical advice and (if they feel it is necessary) refer you to the Child and Adolescent Mental Health Services (CAMHS) for a detailed assessment.

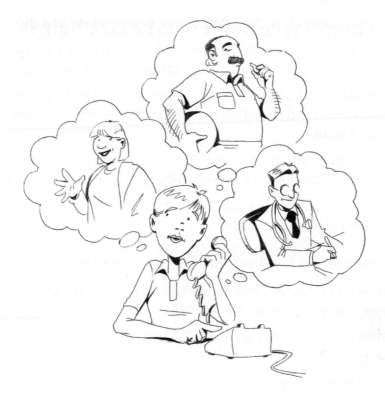

- **Social services**. Social services can be a great source of support for young people and families with particular needs and problems. You can find your local social services office hours' enquiry phone number and a 24-hour emergency phone number in the *Yellow Pages*.

- Your school teacher, head of year, education welfare officer or learning mentor will be best placed to help with school-based problems.

Other organisations you can approach are:

- **ChildLine** (Tel: 0800 1111). This is helpful for children and young people needing advice or just wanting to talk things over. Calls are free and confidential. You can get more information at the ChildLine website (**www.childline.org.uk**).

- **NSPCC**. Adults who are worried about a child can call 0808 800 5000 or visit the NSPCC website (**www.nspcc.org.uk**). Another useful website is www.there4me.com, which is an NSPCC online confidential advice resource for children and young people aged 12 to 16 years who are worried about things such as abuse, bullying, exams, drugs and self-harm. The NSPCC has 24-hour help-lines (for example NSPCC Child Protection Helpline) that you can call to talk things over without the number appearing on house phone bills.

- Local counselling services, such as **Relate** (see **www.relate.org.uk**).

- **Young Minds** provides information and advice for young people with emotional difficulties, their families and friends (see **www.youngminds.org.uk**).

- The **Royal College of Psychiatrists** has fact sheets for family and teachers about common child and young person mental health difficulties (see **www.rcpsych.ac.uk**).

- The **Child Psychotherapy Trust** has produced fact sheets about common child and young person difficulties (see **www.childpsychotherapytrust.org.uk**).

You can buy the following helpful books from local or on-line bookshops or you may find them at your local library:

- *Overcoming Anxiety: A Five Areas Approach* by Chris Williams

- *Think Good – Feel Good: A Cognitive Behaviour Therapy Workbook for Children and Young People* by Paul Stallard

- *Manage Your Mind: The Mental Fitness Guide* by Gillian Butler and Tony Hope

- *Overcoming Depression and Low Mood: A Five Areas Approach* by Chris Williams

- *I'm Not Supposed to Feel Like This: A Christian Self-help Approach to Depression and Anxiety* by Chris Williams, Paul Richards and Ingrid Whitton

- *Overcoming Low Self-Esteem: A Self-Help Guide to Using Cognitive Behavioural Techniques* by Melanie Fennell

- *Mind over Mood* by Christine Padesky and Dennis Greenberger

 www.livinglifetothefull.com and **www.fiveareas.com**

This is a free on-line training course that teaches key life skills by using the same model used in this book. It includes useful additional handouts as well as DVD-based videos to learn key life skills confidentially and for free.

Summary

In this workbook you have:

- Learnt about low mood and depression, and you've had a chance to complete a time line of how your problems have developed

- Learnt how to complete your own Five Areas assessment to monitor how you are feeling

- Learnt how to choose which other course workbooks to use

- Learnt when to get extra help and where to go for it.

Key point

Write down **three things** that went well every day for a week. Stop, think and reflect on this every evening. Why did it go well? Use this to identify any helpful things you have done that you can build on in your life.

A request for feedback

The content of this workbook is updated and improved on a regular basis based on feedback from readers and practitioners. If there are areas in the workbook that you found hard to understand or that seemed unclear, please let us know. However, we don't provide any specific advice on treatment.

To provide feedback please contact us:

Via our website forum: **www.livinglifetothefull.com**

Or by e-mail: **feedback@fiveareas.com**. In your feedback, please can you state which workbook or book you are referring to.

Acknowledgements

We wish to thank all those who have commented on this workbook, especially Keith Chan, Paul Farrand, Steve Yelland, Phil Munroe and Keith Hibbert.

My notes

Overcoming Teenage Low Mood and Depression

A Five Areas Approach

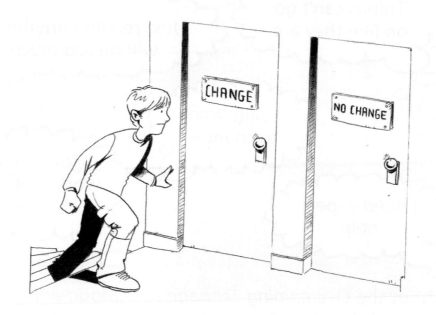

Why bother changing?

Helping you to help yourself
www.livinglifetothefull.com
www.fiveareas.com

Dr Nicky Dummett and Dr Chris Williams

As you start

Are you aware of any of these thoughts?

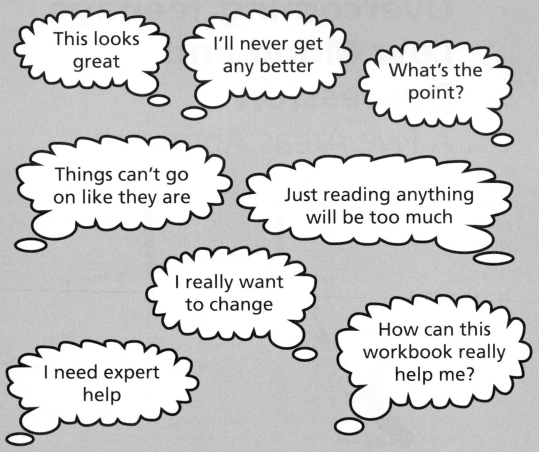

About the *Overcoming Teenage Low Mood and Depression: A Five Areas Approach* workbooks

This course will help you to understand more about how your problems are affecting you. The workbooks will also help you to learn some key skills that you can use to improve how you feel. Many people find the Five Areas Approach helpful because it's practical and focuses on the problems they face now.

Doing this course is also one of the most effective ways of improving low mood.

Everyday language

In particular, this course will provide you with access to the **cognitive behaviour therapy approach** (this is a kind of 'talking treatment', also called CBT for short), by using everyday language that's easy to read and understand.

> ## In this workbook you will:
>
> - Find out how to plan things so you get the most out of the workbook
> - Find out about some common things that can block progress
> - Look at some practical ways to get going and keep going.

Why should you use these workbooks?

Most bookshops have large sections on self-help, and self-help books are often among the top 10 best-selling books. People like to use self-help for all kinds of reasons. The most common reason is that self-help books give us access to key information and skills. **You** – the reader – **are in control**, and you can work on things at the times that suit you rather than your healthcare practitioner. Time and time again, people surprise themselves by the amount of change they can make themselves using a self-help approach.

Next steps

You're most likely to make helpful and positive changes in your life if **you** are in charge of what you read. To get the most from this course, you need to work through it by testing out what you learn in your own life.

 Task

Try to have some protected time every day to think about the things you're learning and the changes you're making in your life.

Write down your immediate reaction to this suggestion.

Completing the tasks set out in each workbook is an important part of trying to change. The day-to-day practice of these tasks will help you get better. In this way you'll bring the workbooks into your everyday life to help you to stop, think and reflect on how you're feeling.

At first, you may think that nothing's changing, but slowly you will notice positive changes. After you've completed each workbook, we'll be encouraging you to judge for yourself how you are doing. For this, we'll be asking you to use the Five Areas model again.

Overcoming blocks to change

One important thing to bear in mind is that our motivation is low during times when we're in a low mood or we're stressed. When we feel low or anxious, it can be hard to make changes. You may:

● Be sleeping poorly

● Have low energy levels

● Find it hard to focus your mind

● Struggle to be motivated to change.

But this can be overcome. In the next section you'll find ideas for different ways in which you can build your motivation to change.

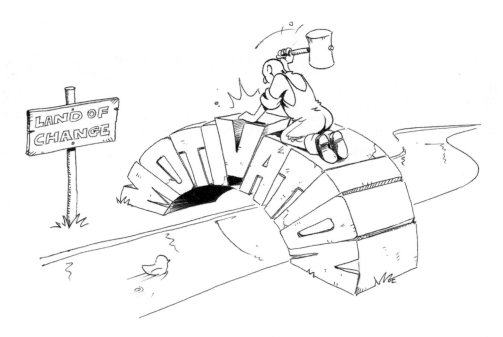

Building your motivation to change
Experiment
Find some time and write to yourself **one of the following two letters**. Try to do this now, before you move on, even if it seems hard to do.

1 **If you aren't quite sure that you are ready for change**. Imagine it's 10 years in the future. Things are going exactly as they are now. Write yourself a letter giving yourself advice and encouragement about why you need to make changes now.

2 **If you've decided that you want change but need some encouragement**. Imagine it's 10 years in the future. You've made important changes in your life and have fully recovered from your depression. Things are much better and you have achieved many of the goals you have set yourself. Write yourself an encouraging letter about why you need to make changes now.

Date: 10 years from now

Dear

Learning to swim

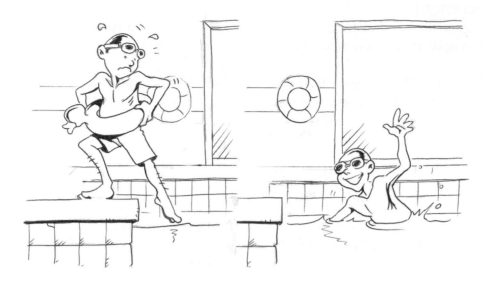

Sometimes it's easy to forget how hard it is to learn new information or skills that you now take for granted. Think about some of the skills you've learnt over the years. For example, if you can swim, think back to your first swimming lesson. You may have struggled a bit at first, yet with practice you learnt the new knowledge and skills that you needed to swim. It may have been hard at that time, but you managed it.

In the same way, you can overcome low mood and tension. It may seem hard at first, but keep practising what you learn.

Key point

Just like swimming you can't expect to get better immediately. So you should use the workbooks in the same way. You may need to start 'at the shallow end' and practise getting better. Pace what you do and don't start by jumping into the deep end.

Having realistic expectations

It would be **untrue** for us to claim that if you use this course you are **guaranteed** results. But what we can say for sure is that the CBT approach has helped thousands of people. And these workbooks teach you about **approaches that have been proved to work**.

We hope you'll feel better in many important ways. But bear in mind that this course also wants to help you to learn some interesting and helpful things along the way.

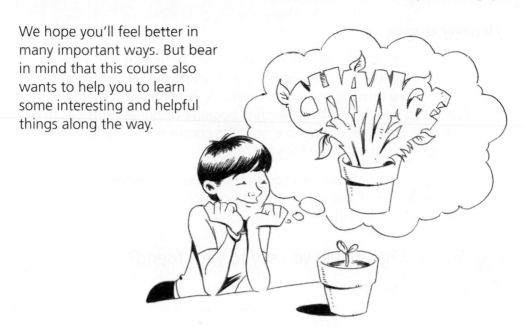

Tackling the things that might stop you using the course

Some things that often seem to cause problems for people in planning to use the workbooks are:

1 **I've no time**

Imagine you had a close friend who was feeling down and distressed. They didn't like how they felt. And you knew that it was affecting them in lots of ways. What advice would you give them if they said, 'I don't have time!'?

… If we can give our friends sensible advice to make some time, could we take that same advice ourselves?

2 **I feel too down to do this**

Sometimes it might not be the right time to do this kind of course, such as when you have severe depression. But remember, you can always plan to come back to it at a later stage if you're finding things too much.

A practical point here is that how much you read this workbook at one time will depend on your concentration. If you find you can't concentrate for long, just try to read one page or even just one paragraph. **Go at a pace you can manage**. If you're feeling like this, you should also discuss the treatment options available to you with your healthcare worker.

3 I'll never change

One of the biggest blocks to getting better is **not believing** that you can change. If you believe that change isn't possible and decide to do nothing, **you may end up missing out** on real benefits. **Remember: change is possible**. Most people find that their first negative response turns out to be incorrect. And they gain much more from the course than they first thought they would. Could this be true for you?

Again, imagine if your friend told you they believed they would never change from a time of low mood. They need encouragement, particularly at the times they believe nothing can change.

Q Again, what would you say to your friend?
Write it down here.

Q If you would offer helpful and positive advice to a friend, then why not offer it to yourself?

But I still don't feel like it!

Sometimes it can be really hard to get going with making the changes needed to improve how we feel. You've made it this far – which is great.

Choose change even if you don't feel like it. Try something small to do first. Put your toes in the water!

Experiment

Even if you have doubts about the course, or about your ability to use it to get better, try giving it a go. In this way you can test it out in your own life. After you've given it a good go, if you still find it doesn't help then that would be a sensible time to try something different.

You might find it useful to come back from time to time to work through this section if you find your motivation to continue the course varies now and then.

How to get the most out of the workbooks

Planning how and when to use the workbooks

Take time to read each workbook you try **at your own pace**. You may find it helpful to set aside a clear time each day to go through the workbooks. But doing this regularly is important – even if it's just a for short time to begin with. So you may find it helpful to actively plan this into your day and diary rather than just 'trying to fit it in some time'.

My plan to use the workbooks

Is reading some of the workbook every day practical for you? If not every day, is every *other* day more realistic? Many people with low mood feel at their worst first thing in the morning. Using the workbooks after lunch or in the late afternoon or in the early evening may be the best time for you.

 When am I going to plan to read the next workbook?

Many people find it helpful to read just one workbook at a time, giving yourself enough time – days, even a week or so. In this way you make sure that you stop, think and reflect by answering the questions as you work through the workbooks.

 How much will I read?

Is this realistic, practical and achievable? (Remember: you know your own life, and its demands and commitments.)

What problems could stop me doing this, and how can I overcome these?

Getting into the mood

Doing something physical can help you get started.

A good way to start to using the workbooks is to do something physical first.

For example, get up and walk around the room, and if there are stairs nearby, walk up and down a few times. Then sit down on a different chair, such as an upright kitchen chair that forces you to sit straight rather than slump back. **Then** start reading the workbook.

Using the workbooks

An important point is that the workbooks are about change. They are **work**books and require some work and effort, but people usually find them easier than they expected.

To help you make this change:

- Have a pen on hand as you read. Try to **answer all the questions** asked.

- **Write down** your own notes in the margins or in the 'My notes' page at the end of the workbook to help you remember information that has been helpful.

- Once you've read through the entire workbook once, **put it on one side** and then **read it again** a few days later. It may be that some parts of the workbook become clearer, or seem more useful, on reading again.

- Use the workbooks to build on the help you receive in other ways. For example, help you get from other helpful reading, talking to friends or family, or self-help organisations and support groups.

- Respond with actions that build on your reading. Try out what you read in the workbooks from the word go.

- Finally, jot down any questions or things you are unsure of as you go along. It will help you remember.

How will I know when I need extra help?

If you find it hard doing the course, don't worry. Just do what you can. However, if things **still** do not seem to be improving, you may need to get extra help. If you have somebody supporting you, discuss what you have been doing with them. Or ask to see your doctor or a mental health worker.

These workbooks aim to help you, and your family and friends, to make changes yourself. But sometimes professional help is needed (perhaps **straight away**). We recommend that ideally, anyone who uses these workbooks has someone to support them in doing it. But there are times when this won't be enough.

You **must get extra help**:

- If you have **severe depression**. For example, if you have a continuing low mood, you're feeling tearful, you aren't eating or drinking much at all, or you feel a big loss of confidence despite your attempts to improve things.

- If you feel like **self-harming** or feel **hopeless** about the future.

- For other concerning **dangerous behaviours**. For example, if you're taking risks or giving threats of harm to others.

- When there is a possibility of immediate or longer-term significant harm or injury to a young person by someone else (that is **physical, emotional or sexual abuse or neglect**).

- If you've **severely withdrawn from life activities**, for example you're missing a lot of school.

There are other situations also when you might need extra help. If either you or the person supporting you is still worried that something else needs to be done, it's important to ask for help. You can do this at least to help you **decide** whether you need more help.

Key point

It's better to ask for help or advice than do nothing.

Summary

In this workbook you have:

- Learnt how to plan things so you get the most out of the workbook
- Learnt about some common things that can block progress
- Learnt some practical ways to get going and keep going.

Let's look at the whole picture again

After you have been putting this workbook into action in your life for a while, rate the size of your problem again in each of the **five areas**.

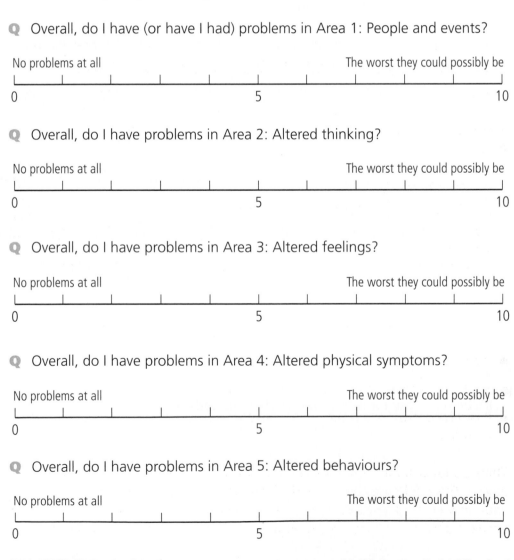

Q Overall, do I have (or have I had) problems in Area 1: People and events?

No problems at all | The worst they could possibly be

0   5   10

Q Overall, do I have problems in Area 2: Altered thinking?

No problems at all | The worst they could possibly be

0   5   10

Q Overall, do I have problems in Area 3: Altered feelings?

No problems at all | The worst they could possibly be

0   5   10

Q Overall, do I have problems in Area 4: Altered physical symptoms?

No problems at all | The worst they could possibly be

0   5   10

Q Overall, do I have problems in Area 5: Altered behaviours?

No problems at all | The worst they could possibly be

0   5   10

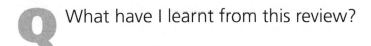 What have I learnt from this review?

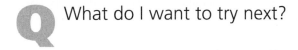 What do I want to try next?

Putting into practice what you have learnt

We know from experience that you'll probably make the most progress if you actually **practise what you've learnt** in each workbook. Each workbook will encourage you to do this by suggesting certain tasks for you to carry out in the following days.

Getting extra support

Everyone is different. Some of us prefer to use the workbooks alone, but others prefer to discuss with someone else what they're learning. This person may be your general practitioner (GP) or other healthcare worker, trusted family member or friend.

Discussing things over with someone else can be helpful because:

● It can help keep you keep on track

● Someone is there to encourage you if you're struggling

● It can be useful to talk through some of the things as you go through the workbooks.

Think about whether someone you know and trust can offer you helpful advice. This might well be a friend of relative. You may want to go through your answers to the workbooks with this person. Or you could keep your answers private and only discuss some of the information you have learnt.

One of the workbooks (*Ideas for families and friends*) is particularly meant for people who are supporting young people using these workbooks.

 www.livinglifetothefull.com

This is a new on-line course, which has been designed to support readers of these workbooks. The on-line teaching sessions are based on this course. They include all the main things covered in the workbooks, plus extra handouts and resources, such as relaxation podcasts.

 www.fiveareas.com

This site contains access to a range of books, handouts, relaxation downloads and other resources using the same approach used in this book.

Other ways to get support

Nowadays, there are many kinds of support for people with low mood and depression. You'll find them listed on pages **28–30** of the *Understanding why I feel as I do* workbook.

A request for feedback

The content of this workbook is updated and improved on a regular basis based on feedback from readers and practitioners. If there are areas in the workbook that you found hard to understand or that seemed unclear, please let us know. However, we don't provide any specific advice on treatment.

To provide feedback please contact us:

 Via our website forum: **www.livinglifetothefull.com**

Or by e-mail: **feedback@fiveareas.com**. In your feedback, please can you state which workbook or book you are referring to.

My notes

PART 2

Making changes

PART 2

Making changes

Overcoming Teenage Low Mood and Depression

A Five Areas Approach

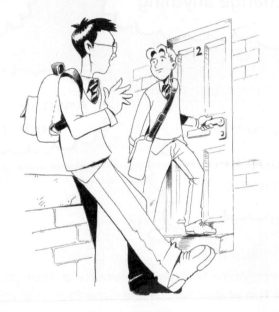

Doing things that make me feel good

Helping you to help yourself

www.livinglifetothefull.com

www.fiveareas.com

Dr Nicky Dummett and Dr Chris Williams

When we feel down or upset, it is often hard to do things. This is because we feel we don't have enough energy and feel tired. And often there is little enjoyment or sense of achievement from what we do. So we start thinking negatively about things.

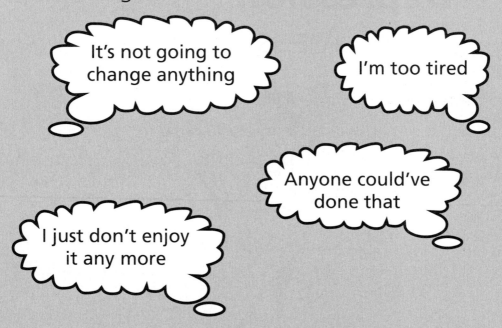

So we often stop doing the things that make us **feel good**. Things we would usually do for **fun** or that help us feel **close** to people or give us a sense of **achievement** can slowly just drop away (for example hobbies, talking with friends or family, exercise, reading books or magazines, meeting or texting friends, or simply relaxing or listening to music).

All this makes us feel even worse.

Often, we focus instead on things we 'have' to do (for example getting unavoidable homework done, doing chores) and just struggling to get by. If our activity levels have reduced a lot, any exercise may feel unusual because we're out of practice or unfit. It can sometimes feel as though everything is just too much effort.

This is sometimes called a **vicious circle of reduced activity**.

Example: Mark's problem

Mark's been feeling down for a few months. He is also struggling with feeling very low in energy. So he's dropped out of the football team a week into the winter term. He'd always enjoyed football and looked forward to it, but this year he has felt 'too tired'. His confidence was also knocked in the first few weeks of term because he missed a few important passes. And once he thought he overhead other people complaining that he was giving chances away. He dropped out of the team without explaining why because he felt too embarrassed. He didn't even talk to his two best friends Jack and Helen because he was feeling so ashamed.

What might Jack and Helen be thinking?

Jack feels hurt and angry and refuses to speak to Mark because he thinks Mark has snubbed him. Helen is worried about Mark but doesn't know how to approach him about this. When she does try to talk to him, Mark thinks that she's going to criticise him and so he reacts defensively, telling her to 'get off my back' and storming out.

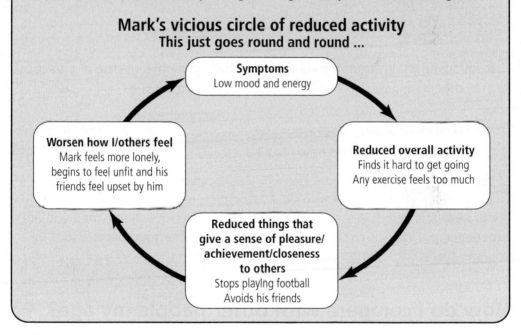

Mark's vicious circle of reduced activity
This just goes round and round ...

- **Symptoms**
  Low mood and energy
- **Reduced overall activity**
  Finds it hard to get going
  Any exercise feels too much
- **Reduced things that give a sense of pleasure/ achievement/closeness to others**
  Stops playing football
  Avoids his friends
- **Worsen how I/others feel**
  Mark feels more lonely, begins to feel unfit and his friends feel upset by him

But the good news is that it's possible to break through the vicious circle.

In this workbook you will:

- Identify any reduced activity in your own life and discover how it has affected you
- Look at some examples of ways of tackling reduced activity
- Practise what you've learnt
- Plan some next steps to build on this improvement.

Are there any things that you've reduced or stopped doing since you started to feel like you do?

1 Have I stopped doing things I used to enjoy as a result of how I feel?

Yes ☐   No ☐   Sometimes ☐

2 Has my reduced activity:

- Removed things from my life that previously gave me a sense of **pleasure**?

Yes ☐   No ☐   Sometimes ☐

- Removed things from my life that previously gave me a sense of **achievement**?

Yes ☐   No ☐   Sometimes ☐

- Removed things from my life that previously gave me a sense of **closeness** to others?

Yes ☐   No ☐   Sometimes ☐

3 Overall, has this worsened how I feel?

Yes ☐   No ☐   Sometimes ☐

If you have answered 'Yes' or 'Sometimes' to all three questions, then you are experiencing a **vicious circle of reduced activity**. The good news is that if you are, this is something you can plan to change.

How do I compare with other people my age?

This is a good question to ask yourself if you're trying to think of activities you may have dropped. Try the Life Activities Scale given here to get you thinking.

Life Activities Scale

Put a cross on each line below to show how much of each of these activities you do compared with what you did before you felt unwell. It may help to also consider how much you do compared with most people your age. On the scale 0 per cent means 'I don't do this at all' and 100 per cent means 'I do just as much of this as most people my age'.

1 Keeping up with my self-care (washing, dressing, eating properly)

0%   50%   100%

2 Getting up and going to bed at about the same time as most people

0%   50%   100%

3 Hobbies and things I do to relax or enjoy myself

0%   50%   100%

4 Keeping up with homework and other things I need to get done

0%   50%   100%

5 Getting out and about (out of the house, shopping, travelling)

0%   50%   100%

6 Getting to and staying at school or college

0%   50%   100%

7 Spending time socialising with family

0%   50%   100%

8 Spending time socialising with friends

0%   50%   100%

Choosing some activities to focus on to start with means that you are actively choosing at first **not** to focus on other areas. These could possibly be the things that were getting you down. Setting clear targets will help you to focus on how to make the changes you need to get better.

What do I want to focus on first?

 Task

Think of your answers to the Life Activities Scale and write the things you've stopped doing below.

1 Things I have reduced or stopped doing that gave me a sense of **pleasure**:

2 Things I have reduced or stopped doing that gave me a sense of **achievement** – the sort of things I would say 'well done' to someone else:

3 Things I have reduced or stopped doing that gave me a sense of **closeness** to other people:

How do I work out what other things make me feel good?

Keeping an activity diary

In the activity diary on page **57** write everything you do for four days. There is another copy of this activity diary at the back of this workbook for you to photocopy so that you have enough. This will help you begin to work out what things have made you feel better. Record **everything** that you do (for example getting dressed, talking on the phone, using the internet, doing some homework, shopping, washing your hair, helping with the washing up). Also include the times when you are watching television, having a bath or resting, etc.

My activity diary

Rate **each** activity you did for:

1 Any **pleasure** it gave you, how much you **enjoyed** doing it (from 0 = no pleasure to 10 = a lot of pleasure)

2 How much of an **achievement** you feel it was (from 0 = no sense of achievement to 10 = a huge sense of achievement)

3 How much of a feeling of **closeness** to other people it gave you (from 0 = no sense of closeness to 10 = a big sense of closeness)

Day	Activity (what I was doing)	How long I did it for (in minutes)	Pleasure (0 to 10)	Achievement (0 to 10)	Closeness (0 to 10)
7–8 am					
8–9 am					
9–10 am					
10–11 am					
11–12 pm					
12–1 pm					
1–2 pm					

Day	Activity (what I was doing)	How long I did it for (in minutes)	Pleasure (0 to 10)	Achievement (0 to 10)	Closeness (0 to 10)
2–3 pm					
3–4 pm					
4–5 pm					
5–6 pm					
6–7 pm					
7–8 pm					
8–9 pm					
9–10 pm					
10–11 pm					
11–12 am					
Later					

Key point

Try filling in one of the spare activity diaries in the back of this workbook for a time **well before** you started to feel down or stressed (say a year or so back). This may help you see what other helpful activities you have stopped.

Here is part of Mark's activity diary. It shows that even though he's doing less than usual (he's no longer playing football), he's still doing some things that help him feel better. **Once he knows this** he can plan to do more of them.

Day	Activity (what I was doing)	How long I did it for (in minutes)	Pleasure (0 to 10)	Achievement (0 to 10)	Closeness (0 to 10)
7–8 am	Woke up, got dressed and had breakfast alone, watching TV	50 min	3	2	0
8–9 am	Got ready for school and walked there alone	40 min	3	6	0
9–10 am	Registration and assembly with my class First class starts (maths)	15 min 45 min	5	5	5
10–11 am	In class doing French – did some work in a small discussion group	90 mins	6	5	7
11–12 pm	Played cards in break Classes	20 min 40 min	7 5	4 4	8 4
12–1 pm	Lunch and sat alone	45 min	4	3	0

Mark has discovered that he feels the most pleasure when he is playing cards with his friends. In fact, he tends to feel generally **happier when he's with other people**, and has a sense of closeness (for example playing cards, in assembly, in the small group discussion). His biggest sense of achievement tends to be when he gets to school in the first place – even when he hasn't looked forward to it, and also when he does things with others in class.

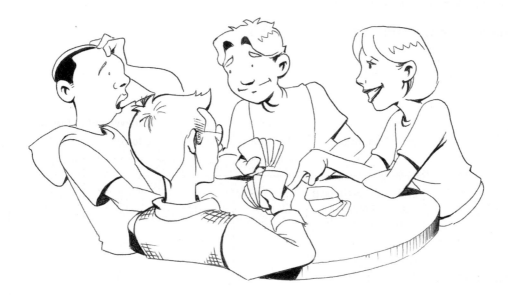

Choosing a target

From Mark's activity diary, a clear target for Mark to work on might be to boost the things that give him a sense of closeness and pleasure – for example eating with others at home, seeing if there is anyone he could walk to school with, and seeing if he can boost the times he meets others in breaks and over lunch. Another good idea would be to do things that give a sense of achievement.

Look at your activity diary to see what has given you a sense of pleasure or achievement or closeness to other people. You may be surprised at what you discover! Building in a time each day to think about and remember helpful things can boost your mood too. Use the following checklist to discover any other helpful things you may have stopped.

As a result of how I feel, am I:	Tick here if you have noticed this (even if just sometimes)
Stopping or reducing doing hobbies or interests such as reading or other things I used to enjoy or did to relax?	☐
Going out or meeting up with friends less than usual?	☐
Eating poorly (for example eating less food in general or tending to eat more 'junk' food)?	☐
Exercising so little that any exercise feels an effort?	☐
No longer taking up exciting opportunities or 'living life to the full'?	☐
Not always answering the phone or the door when people visit?	☐
Leaving letters, e-mails or texts unopened or not replying to them because of a lack of energy or interest in actively dealing with them?	☐
Paying less attention to my self-care or personal hygiene (for example washing less, being less bothered about my appearance, leaving clothes on for longer, not shaving or combing my hair)?	☐
If you have a religious faith: reduced or stopped reading my holy book, praying or going to my place of worship?	☐

 Task

Have I reduced or stopped doing any other things?

Write them down here:

More good news ...

All you have to do to feel better is **start doing** more of the things that make you feel better! This doesn't just mean doing more jobs. Instead it means **doing more things that give you** a sense of pleasure, achievement or closeness to others.

So how can you slowly start to get more of these helpful things back into your daily routine in a way that isn't too much extra effort? The trick is to try building things back into your life **one at a time**, rather than all at once. Choose which you want to do first. What activity has given you most pleasure, sense of achievement or closeness?

By choosing and planning just one thing to boost fun, closeness or achievement you can slowly plan more and more of these activities into your life. Let's start by planning the first thing you want to do. You can then move on to plan more and more things that give you a boost.

My first step

 Task

Write **one activity** you want to build back into your life here. Remember that this should be something you have stopped doing and **not doing it has worsened** how you feel.

The key to start doing your chosen activity again is to use a **step-by-step** approach. Break the activity down into small steps so no step seems too large. In this way you can use this activity to **slowly and steadily tackle** your problems and rebuild your confidence.

The **first step** simply needs to be something that gets you moving in the right direction. Ask yourself – is this first step:

- Realistic and achievable so that I am likely to succeed?
- Not so scary that I can't face doing it?
- Still big enough to move me forward?

My first step will be:

Key point

You need to have a clear **overall plan** that will help you decide exactly **what** steps you're going to do to build up your target activity, and roughly **when** you're going to do them. In this way you can plan how long it will take and to think of any problems that are likely to arise.

 Task

Now write down exactly **how** you're going to carry out the first step of your plan and **when** you are going to do it. Also write down ways of tackling any possible blocks that might get in your way.

Ask yourself the following **questions for effective change**.

 ## Is this first step one that:

- Will be **useful** for understanding or changing how I am?

  Yes ☐ No ☐

- Is a **specific** task so that I will know when I have done it?

  Yes ☐ No ☐

- Is realistic, practical and achievable?

  Yes ☐   No ☐

- Makes clear what I am going to do and when I am going to do it?

  Yes ☐   No ☐

- Is an activity that won't be easily blocked or prevented by practical problems?

  Yes ☐   No ☐

- Will help me to learn useful things even if it doesn't work out perfectly?

  Yes ☐   No ☐

You should've answered 'Yes' to all of the questions. Remember to build into your plan what you will do if the plan doesn't fully succeed.

Q What will I do if this step doesn't fully succeed?

Write down what you can do instead here.

And now … **Just do it!**

Decide when you'll do the first step of your plan (for example during the next week). Write in your activity diary **exactly** when you'll do it so it's clear when you will do it. Now see how it goes!

Key point

Remember that as you carry out the plan you are undermining your old doubts and fears by **acting against** them. Pay attention to the thoughts you have before, during and afterwards about what will happen.

My review

Q How did it go?

📌 **Task**

Write down what happened here:

Q Did the step-by-step plan work for you?

Yes ☐   No ☐

Q Did it help improve things?

Yes ☐   No ☐

Q Did making these changes make it worse for you in any way?

Yes ☐   No ☐

Q What have I learnt from doing this?

Q What is the next step?

Learning from my review

If things didn't go quite as you hoped, write here any helpful lessons or information you have learned. Choosing realistic targets for change is important.

Q Was I being too ambitious or unrealistic when I chose this target?

Q Did something unexpected happen, for example something didn't happen as planned, or someone reacted in an unexpected way?

Q How could I make things different next time I tackle the problem?

Example: Mark's first step

Mark has planned to run for 15 minutes after school on Monday as a first step to getting back to running regularly (he used to enjoy it and used to get a huge sense of achievement from running). In case things go wrong, he has decided he **will** run even if he doesn't feel on the night that it's a good idea. He's also agreed with his mum that she will remind him to run if he doesn't get on with it.

Mark gets home from school on Monday evening and feels very tired. He thinks 'What's the point? I can't believe I will even be **able** to run.' He believes this 80 per cent and feels quite down. He thinks back to his plan and decides to do what he had planned anyway. He gets changed before his mother has a chance to remind him to go out. He goes for his run, and half way through it he realises how good he feels. Although the running was difficult for the first few minutes, he is surprised to find he feels more energetic and positive about things quite quickly.

He rates his level of pleasure, achievement and closeness afterwards as:

- Pleasure: 90 per cent
- Achievement: 90 per cent
- Closeness: 10 per cent. I know my mum would have encouraged me if I needed. I also mean to run with other people in future.

Overall, Mark realises that he **has** gained a lot of pleasure and a definite sense of achievement from the run and that his predictions about how it would go wrong were unfounded.

Example: Mark's review

Overall, that went really well. I did find it difficult getting going. I almost talked myself out of it, but it was good to have planned things so I knew my mum would say something if I didn't go.

Even though I felt tired, and had some doubts before going about whether I could run at all, when I got going things went really well. I think 15 minutes was about right. I was tempted to go for a bit longer, but I decided to stick to the plan. It's just as well because I felt a bit achy in the shower afterwards. I definitely feel it lifted me. I'm looking forward to doing this again soon.

Planning the next steps

Do

- Continue to plan to alter only **one area of your target activity** at a time.

- Remember to continue breaking down the problem into **smaller parts** that each builds towards your eventual goal. There can be as many or as few steps as you want in your plan.

- Produce a plan to slowly alter what you do in an effective way.

- Be realistic in your goals.

- Use the 'questions for effective change' (pages **63–4**) to help plan each step.

- Write down your plan in detail so that you can start in that week.

- If you find any step too difficult, **go back a stage and regain your confidence**. Then, decide on a different next step that is not quite so difficult. Repeat this step successfully several times before trying again with the step you found too difficult.

Don't

- Choose something that is too ambitious a target to do next.

- Try to make too many changes in your life all at once.

- Be very negative and think 'nothing can be done'. Instead, try to experiment to find out if this negative thinking is true or helpful.

- Try to move too quickly from one step to the next. Instead, make sure you repeatedly succeed at each step first.

Key information

Most problems can be overcome using this approach. Remember, the commonest reasons for a plan not to work are if you are **too ambitious** or if you allow yourself to believe that change is impossible.

Practical hints and tips for boosting activity

- Photocopy the blank diary at the end of this workbook to plan your activities. Each week you should include a range of things that give you a sense of **pleasure**, **achievement** and **closeness** to other people.

- Use your activity diary to plan to do something **for yourself** each day. For example, reading, having a bath, listening to music, having a little treat or time for yourself – even if just a little each day.

- Is there something creative you've wanted to do like start playing an instrument, or play in a band or do some kind of art work?

- Get in contact with people you **like** – by text, letter, e-mail or phone.

  Talk and listen more. Do things together. Don't overly focus on just one relationship.

  The *Being assertive* workbook and *Building relationships* workbook can help you with this. If you have felt isolated for a long time and it's difficult to think of someone you might contact, then switch to a problem-solving approach. Work through the *Practical problem solving* workbook with this in mind.

- Consider taking up something you value, especially something that gives you a sense of purpose. For example, voluntary work, helping tidy a local park, or helping a community or religious organisation. Could you join an after-school activity or club if you've enjoyed that in the past?

- **Write down some goals** in a notebook at the start of the week and take satisfaction as you tick them off at the end of the week. Also, at the end of the week write down any other things that you've achieved. Make sure your **goals are realistic** and really can be managed within that week.

- **Exercise** can have an important and positive effect on many aspects of your life. An increase in exercise will help boost your mood, make you feel healthier and help you sleep better. Generally people are recognising the benefits of exercise. Is there a team sport you have enjoyed before or would like to try? You can find out more about how to do this in the *Using exercise to boost how I feel* workbook.

Key point

Remember – small steps at a time!

Don't try to change more than one thing at a time. Break anything you try into small, 'do-able' steps. These are only ideas to get you thinking – you don't have to do all of them!

Summary

In this workbook you have:

- Discovered how lowered activity affects our lives
- Identified any reduced activity in your own life and thought about its effect on you
- Learnt how to record your current activity levels
- Seen examples of ways of overcoming reduced activity
- Practised this approach yourself to make slow, steady changes to your life
- Planned some next steps to build on this improvement.

Let's look at the whole picture again

After you've been putting this workbook into action in your life for a while, rate the size of your problems again in each of the **five areas**.

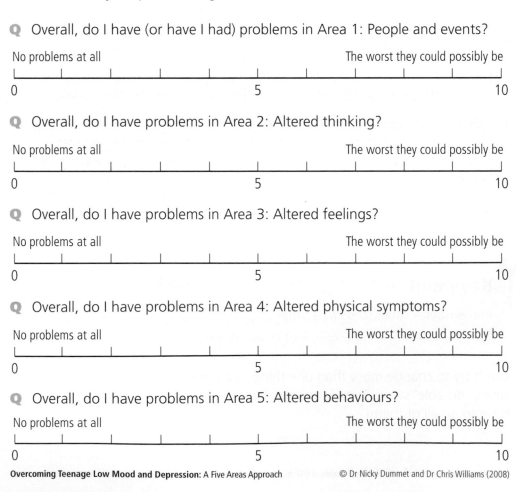

Q Overall, do I have (or have I had) problems in Area 1: People and events?

No problems at all   The worst they could possibly be

0   5   10

Q Overall, do I have problems in Area 2: Altered thinking?

No problems at all   The worst they could possibly be

0   5   10

Q Overall, do I have problems in Area 3: Altered feelings?

No problems at all   The worst they could possibly be

0   5   10

Q Overall, do I have problems in Area 4: Altered physical symptoms?

No problems at all   The worst they could possibly be

0   5   10

Q Overall, do I have problems in Area 5: Altered behaviours?

No problems at all   The worst they could possibly be

0   5   10

What have I learnt from this review?

 What do I want to try next?

Putting into practice what you have learnt
 Task

Make and do some action plans over the next few weeks to tackle your reduced activity. If you have problems just do what you can. You may surprise yourself!

A request for feedback

The content of this workbook is updated and improved on a regular basis based on feedback from readers and practitioners. If there are areas in the workbook that you found hard to understand or that seemed unclear, please let us know. However, we don't provide any specific advice on treatment.

To provide feedback please contact us:

 Via our website forum: **www.livinglifetothefull.com**

Or by e-mail: **feedback@fiveareas.com**. In your feedback, please can you state which workbook or book you are referring to.

My notes

My activity diary

Write out or photocopy this page for further use, or download it for free from **www.fiveareas.com**.

Rate **each** activity you did for:

1 Any **pleasure** it gave you and how much you **enjoyed** doing it (from 0 = no pleasure to 10 = a lot of pleasure).

2 How much of an **achievement** you feel it was (from 0 = no sense of achievement to 10 = a big sense of achievement).

3 How much of a feeling of **closeness** to other people it gave you (from 0 = no sense of closeness to 10 = a big sense of closeness).

Day	Activity (what I was doing)	How long I did it for (in minutes)	Pleasure (0 to 10)	Achievement (0 to 10)	Closeness (0 to 10)
7–8 am					
8–9 am					
9–10 am					
10–11 am					
11–12 pm					
12–1 pm					
1–2 pm					
2–3 pm					
3–4 pm					
4–5 pm					
5–6 pm					
6–7 pm					
7–8 pm					
8–9 pm					
9–10 pm					
10–11 pm					
11–12 am					
Later					

Overcoming Teenage Low Mood and Depression

A Five Areas Approach

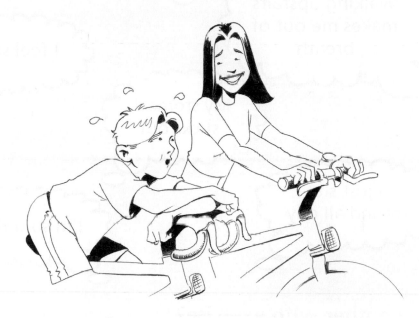

Using exercise to boost how I feel

Helping you to help yourself
www.livinglifetothefull.com
www.fiveareas.com

Dr Nicky Dummett and Dr Chris Williams

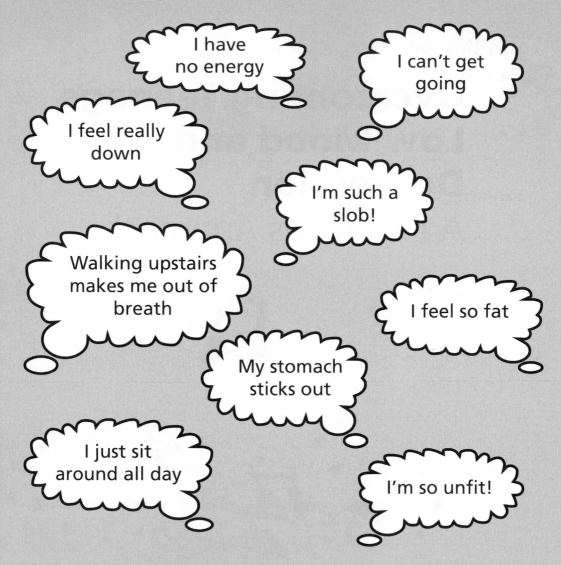

Why bother with exercise?

Our emotions, thinking, behaviour, relationships, life situation and body all affect each other. They are all connected.

Increasing **your physical activity levels can boost how you feel** mentally as well as physically. We often forget to exercise when we feel unwell or it seems too hard. Think about a time when you have had a bad cold. Besides a runny nose and a sore throat, did you feel like just being quiet, and feel fed-up and down as well?

Now think back to a time when you exercised – such as riding a bike, playing football, swimming. Some people find that they often get a **mental 'high'** after exercise.

In this workbook you will:

- See how exercise can boost your mood

- Learn how to exercise to reduce your tension and anxiety

- See how to improve your self-esteem by becoming physically fitter.

Why exercise may be good for you

We often forget to exercise when we feel unwell or it seems too hard. Exercise can now be 'prescribed' by doctors as part of treatment for depression.

- Exercise can be fun if you choose something that you have previously liked doing.

- It gives **you** control to plan things at your own pace.

- It can help you structure and plan your day – rather than just staying in and being inactive.

- It can boost your social life. Doing things with others such as a step class, going for a run with your friends, playing football or going for a swim can help you meet others who share interests.

- It really is a win–win situation.

Possible downsides of exercise

You may have a few problems when thinking about boosting your physical activity.

- You can expect to notice aching muscles to begin with!

- There can be a cost for some activities (for example for using a gym or swimming pool).

How planned exercise can help you feel better

Experiment

You'll need less than 15 minutes to do this experiment. The aim is to test if even a small amount of exercise affects how you feel overall.

Before you start think of a physical activity that you can do. This should be something:

- That can be done in just 5–10 minutes to start with

- That is realistic, bearing in mind how you are physically at the moment

- That you know you can do and doesn't push you. Please choose something that doesn't involve vigorous exercise.

Key point

This isn't asking you to do a workout. You don't need to get changed, work up a sweat or even do warm-up exercises.

Here's an example: Walk up and down a flight of stairs three to four times. Take some rest if you get out of breath.

Other things you could try are stretching your body, jogging slowly on the spot or walking round the block at a reasonable pace. Remember not to overdo it. Aim to do something that gets your heart rate up and gets you moving **without being excessive**. Remember, any benefits can be boosted even more by planning to do activities that are fun or sociable.

If you think you're physically unwell you can always check this with your doctor first, if you have any worries.

Doing your planned exercise

So you've chosen what to do. **Before you start** put a cross on the two lines below to show how you feel right now.

How I feel now

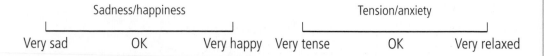

Sadness/happiness

Very sad OK Very happy

Tension/anxiety

Very tense OK Very relaxed

Now do your 5–10 minutes exercise. Remember you can stop for a rest if you feel this is too long for you.

Your review

Immediately afterwards please rate your mood again.

How I feel after my exercise

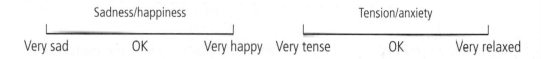

Sadness/happiness

Very sad OK Very happy

Tension/anxiety

Very tense OK Very relaxed

Next: stop, think and reflect

Have a look at your scores before and after.

 Task

Q Did you notice any changes? Write down any changes you noticed in your thoughts, in your mental energy, in how positive you feel and in your ability to think clearly.

Q How did you feel during the task? Write down what you felt (tension, anger, stress, sadness, happiness, enthusiasm).

Q How did you feel physically? Write down what you felt (relaxed or tense, jittery, tired, achy, ready for more).

Q Write down any other changes you noticed.

Q Overall, do you think you might benefit from planning in some exercise into your life as part of your own 'mental fitness' package?

Yes ☐ No ☐ Sometimes ☐

Yes, but …

There are often lots of things in life that we know are good for us, but we don't do them. This is true for most people.

Tackling the simple blocks

Often the biggest problems are simple ones:

- We just aren't in the habit of doing exercise.
- We want to get into the habit but it proves hard. For example, it's easy for us to talk ourselves out of it.

It is a common problem.

Many of us see exercise as too hard or boring, too expensive, taking too much time – or all of these!

What thoughts block you from doing exercise?

But you don't have to make a drastic lifestyle change. Small changes can **all** make a positive difference. Find a way to make this easier for yourself, for example fitting it into what you already do each day.

Remember it's important to **warm up to avoid muscle pulls, aches and strains**. *Using good techniques and the right equipment, clothing and shoes is also important.*

Making a clear plan that works for you

People are often amazed at how empowering, energising and good it can feel when they get into the habit of exercising as part of their regular daily routine.

- Choose something that gets you going physically. Build up the amount of exercise slowly in a gradual and planned way.

- Don't throw yourself into things too quickly (or start too slowly). **Pacing is the key**.

- Many people find that doing exercise towards the start of the day helps them to 'get going'. Try to avoid exercising just before going to bed as this can unhelpfully affect your sleep.

- Look to do this with help. Plan to exercise with a friend.

- If you've signed up to the **www.livinglifetothefull.com** course you can get short **monthly e-mail reminders** to help keep you on track. This course is free and you can cancel at any time. (Please note the course doesn't offer advice on an individual basis.)

Planning when and how to exercise

Exercising on a regular basis – even if it is just a short time to begin with – is important. It is often helpful to actively plan this into your day and diary rather than just 'trying to fit it in some time'. You may find the following **planning task** helpful in making this regular commitment.

My plan to use exercise to help me feel better

Q **What** am I going to do?

(Remember to choose something that is possible, realistic and achievable. Preferably choose something that is fun. Consider planning in some exercise that has a social aspect at least once a week, for example a step class or going for a run or walk with some friends. Remember exercise doesn't need to cost lots of money. Exercise videos and DVDs are available for a small weekly charge at your local library. Or you could walk to your local shop each time instead of taking the bus or being driven.)

Q **When** am I going to plan to do some exercise?

(Think about whether doing some exercise every day is practical for you. If it is, what time of day would be best for you? If you can't manage it every day then how about just once or twice a week? You can always build on this later.)

Q **How much** exercise will I do?

(Be realistic – think about your current level of fitness, health and motivation. If you have doubts about your health, please discuss this with your doctor.)

Q Is this **realistic**, practical and achievable?

(Remember you know your own life, and its demands and commitments.)

Q What problems could stop me doing exercise and how can I overcome them?

(For example, school, college or work deadlines, money, or having the kit you need.)

Keeping on track

Once you have created your exercise plan it is **important to keep on track**. This means setting yourself goals and reviewing your progress. In this way you can make changes if things aren't going well.

My plan for the next few weeks

(Think about short-term, medium-term and long-term changes.)

Q What are you going to do?

1

2

3

Q How will you try to make sure that you carry out your plan?

Q When are you going to do it?

Q What can stop this happening

(What problems might there be, and how can you overcome them? What might interfere with your plan?)

Date of my next review (review your plan monthly, set aside a time to do this). Put the date into your diary.

Summary

In this workbook you have:

- Learnt how exercise can boost how you feel
- Learnt about the benefits and 'side effects' of exercise
- Found out about ways of planning exercise into your life in a paced way.

Let's look at the whole picture again

After you have been putting this workbook into action in your life for a while, rate the size of your problems again in each of the **five areas**.

Q Overall, do I have (or have I had) problems in Area 1: People and events?

No problems at all   The worst they could possibly be

0   5   10

Q Overall, do I have problems in Area 2: Altered thinking?

No problems at all   The worst they could possibly be

0   5   10

Q Overall, do I have problems in Area 3: Altered feelings?

No problems at all   The worst they could possibly be

0   5   10

Q Overall, do I have problems in Area 4: Altered physical symptoms?

No problems at all   The worst they could possibly be

0   5   10

Q Overall, do I have problems in Area 5: Altered behaviours?

No problems at all   The worst they could possibly be

0   5   10

What have I learnt from this review?

 What do I want to try next?

Putting things into practice

Read this workbook again. Make a plan for your own exercise and try to stick to it.

Other ways to get support

- Your general practitioner (GP) may be able to refer you to an exercise class.

- Look out for classes at your local swimming pool or gym.

- Think about tennis, badminton or walking classes.

- Find out more: the Mental Health Foundation provides useful information on its website about exercise and mood (see **www.mentalhealth.org.uk**).

- Do it with a friend! Plan to do exercise with a friend, classmate or colleague.

 Do the on-line module about healthy living at
www.livinglifetothefull.com

My notes

Overcoming Teenage Low Mood and Depression

A Five Areas Approach

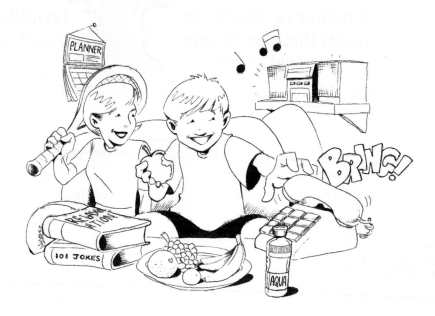

Helpful things we do

Helping you to help yourself
www.livinglifetothefull.com
www.fiveareas.com

Dr Nicky Dummett and Dr Chris Williams

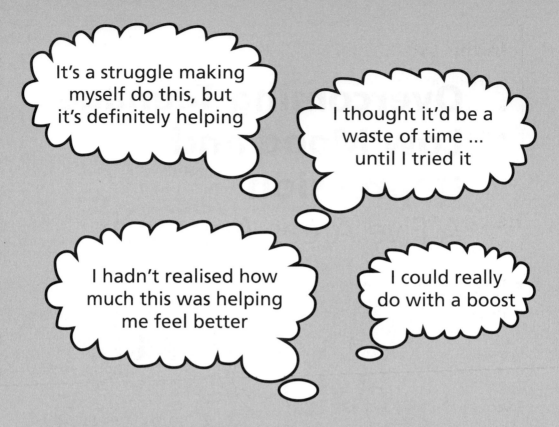

When we feel low or depressed, **it is normal** to try to do things to help us feel better, **but** the things we try can be **helpful** or **unhelpful**.

Key information

Unhelpful behaviours actually backfire and make things worse, perhaps not immediately, but often later. If you're wondering if something you are doing to try to make you feel better may actually be unhelpful, read the workbook *Unhelpful things we do*.

We also often drop helpful things we've been doing as we've lost faith in them. Also everything may seem like just too much of an effort.

In this workbook you will:

- Learn about helpful ways of responding to low mood and depression

- Think about other people's helpful behaviours

- Decide which behaviours help **you** – and plan how to build these back into your life.

Helpful behaviours

Helpful behaviours include:

- Things you can do yourself

- Things you can do with others.

Different things help different people, but there are things that can help most people.

Some of these good ideas are:

- Keeping doing things that bring a sense of **pleasure**, **achievement** or **closeness** to others, for example meeting friends, joining a group (see the workbook *Doing things that make me feel good*)

- Keeping doing the everyday things that most people your age do as part of normal life (see the workbook *Doing things that make me feel good*, Life Activities Scale, page **55**)

- Talking and receiving support from family or friends

- Checking the internet, using self-help materials, attending a self-help group or talking to your doctor to find out more about overcoming low mood

- Challenging anxious thoughts by stopping, thinking and reflecting rather than **always** accepting them as true.

You will also get more ideas of helpful behaviours from other workbooks in this course.

Am I already doing anything that helps?

Checklist of helpful behaviours

Am I ...	Tick here if you do this (even if just sometimes)
Being good to myself? Eating regularly and healthily – taking time to enjoy the food	☐
Keeping up with the daily life activities we all need to keep feeling good? (See the workbook *Doing things that make me feel good*, Life Activities Scale, page 55.) For example, going to bed and getting up at sensible times	☐
Doing things that bring a sense of pleasure, achievement or closeness to others? For example, meeting friends, joining a group (see the workbook *Doing things that make me feel good*)	☐
Doing things for fun/pleasure? For example, hobbies, listening to music, having a nice bath	☐
Sharing worries with trusted friends and family? And giving myself permission to get help from other people	☐
Seeking out other helpful sources of information and support? For example, using the internet or attending a self-help group	☐
Socialising at a level I can cope with? For example, by telephone, e-mail or going out – giving yourself the chance to enjoy being with people and feeling close	☐
Pacing myself – and letting others know I am doing this? For example, telling family and friends I am planning to do things bit by bit	☐
Stopping, thinking and reflecting on things rather than jumping to conclusions? And letting upsetting thoughts 'just be' rather than constantly mulling them over? (See the workbook *Noticing and changing negative thinking* for more help with this)	☐
Keeping as active as I can? For example, doing exercise, going for walks, swimming or going to a gym	☐
Using my sense of humour to cope?	☐
Planning time for me as well as for others?	☐
Taking any prescribed medication regularly and as prescribed?	☐
Using coping responses that work, such as relaxation techniques to deal with feelings of tension? (See **www.livinglifetothefull.com** and **www.fiveareas.com**)	☐

Task

Write down any **helpful things** you have done or **are still doing** here.

Ask yourself about each one you've written about above:

1 Is this definitely helpful in the short-term **and** longer-term for me?

Yes ☐   No ☐   Sometimes ☐

2 Overall has this improved how I and others feel?

Yes ☐   No ☐   Sometimes ☐

If you have answered 'Yes' or 'Sometimes' to these questions, you are responding in some helpful ways. Well done! Building more of these helpful behaviours into your life is an important part of getting better.

Things other people can do

Family and friends can often offer support and a listening ear. So when we're feeling down it can be helpful and encouraging to have family and friends around us. But **too much** help from others can be frustrating or even undermine our confidence in ourselves. What's needed is a **balanced supportive relationship**.

You need to give others a clear message about what you do (or do not) want or need (see the *Being assertive* workbook for more ideas about this). Also, you might want to try reading the workbook *Ideas for families and friends* to think about the things others do that are helpful and what isn't helpful for you.

If you are clear that something someone is doing **has** been helpful, tell them this. Ask if they can do more of it. Think of anyone else who could do it too.

Step 7: Review your learning

Example: Helen reviews her plan

That went really well. I felt we really connected — and felt very close to Mum. It was good to see that she really wanted to do this. She looked like she enjoyed it. I did too.

Write down your own review of what happened with your plan.

Ask yourself:

- Was my approach successful?

  Yes ☐   No ☐

- Did it help improve things?

  Yes ☐   No ☐

- Did I have any problems with using this approach?

  Yes ☐   No ☐

What have I learnt from doing this?

If things didn't go quite as you hoped, write here any helpful lessons or information you have learnt. Remember that choosing realistic targets for change is important.

Q Did I choose a target that required too much from me or my family or friends?

Q Did something unexpected happen, for example things didn't happen as planned, or someone reacted in an unexpected way?

Q How could I make things different the next time I tackle this target?

Q Did your plan help you to completely solve your problem?(Don't worry if it didn't – or if it only helped a little. Most people need to think of more ways to build other helpful behaviours.)

Planning the next steps

Now that you have reviewed how your first step went, the next step is to plan another change to build on the first one. You need to think about your **short-term, medium-term** and **longer-term** targets – where you think you want to be in a week's time, a few months' time or a year's time.

Key point

You will need to slowly build on what you have done in **a step-by-step way**.

So you can now choose to:

- Focus on the same helpful behaviour but plan to increase it further
- Or select a new helpful behaviour to work on
- Or stick at the target you have achieved.

For each choice, think about what the pros (advantages) will be and what the cons (disadvantages) may be for you.

Choosing a next helpful behaviour

If you've decided to work on a new helpful behaviour, you can look at the checklist of helpful behaviours on page **92** again to choose another one.

Key point

Create your own clear **longer-term plan** and then work on it one step at a time. This will help you to practise and reinforce your skills in creating such a plan.

Do

- Be realistic. Plan to do **only** one or two new key helpful behaviours over the next week. Don't try to do too much too soon and burn out.
- Make a **longer-term plan** to slowly change what you do, for example over the next six weeks.
- Quiz yourself to check that the change is well planned.
- Write down your plan in detail, so that you'll know exactly what to do.

Don't

- Try to start to change too many things all at once.
- Choose something that is too big a next step.
- Be negative and think, 'Nothing can be done. What's the point? It's a waste of time'. **Try things out to test** whether this negative thinking really is right and whether it really does help you.

Your new action plan

Plan **what** you will do and **when** you will do it.

Q   What will I try in the next few weeks?

Q   What will I try in the next few months?

Q   What will I try over the next year?

Learn from what happens so that you can keep putting into practice what you have learnt. By doing this, you will be able to bring about slow but steady changes in a planned, step-by-step way. You'll build your confidence again and increase your control over any unhelpful behaviours.

Keeping going

Again, remember to keep putting into practice what you learn over the next few weeks. Don't try to solve every problem you face all at once, but plan out what to do at a pace that's right for you. Build changes one step at a time.

Summary

In this workbook you have:

- Learnt about helpful ways of responding to low mood and depression
- Learnt some useful ways to increase helpful behaviours
- Practised a step-by-step approach to plan an increase in helpful behaviour.

Let's look at the whole picture again

After you have put this workbook into action in your life for a while, rate the size of your problems again in each of the **five areas**.

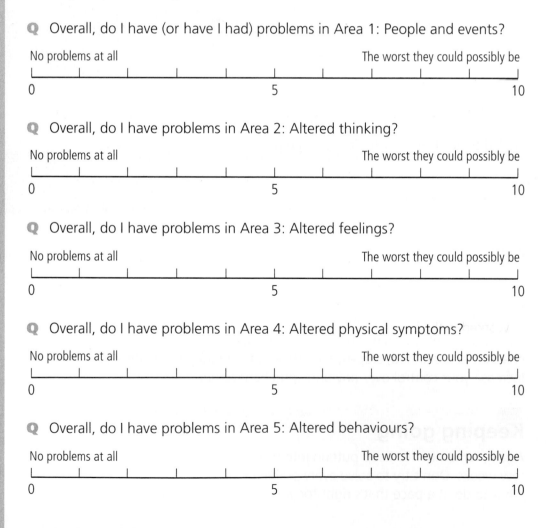

Q Overall, do I have (or have I had) problems in Area 1: People and events?

No problems at all   The worst they could possibly be

0   5   10

Q Overall, do I have problems in Area 2: Altered thinking?

No problems at all   The worst they could possibly be

0   5   10

Q Overall, do I have problems in Area 3: Altered feelings?

No problems at all   The worst they could possibly be

0   5   10

Q Overall, do I have problems in Area 4: Altered physical symptoms?

No problems at all   The worst they could possibly be

0   5   10

Q Overall, do I have problems in Area 5: Altered behaviours?

No problems at all   The worst they could possibly be

0   5   10

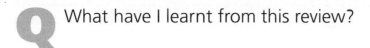 What have I learnt from this review?

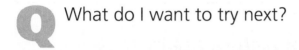 What do I want to try next?

Other ways of getting support and information

Think about how to involve:

- **Yourself** – because ultimately it's down to you to plan to change your altered behaviours

- Friends you trust

- Your family

- Your teacher

- Your general practitioner (GP) or other healthcare practitioners you have worked with.

You can also read the section 'Getting extra help' in the *Understanding why I feel as I do* workbook.

 Do the online module at **www.livinglifetothefull.com** or use the support forum there to swap ideas and encouragement.

My notes

Overcoming Teenage Low Mood and Depression

A Five Areas Approach

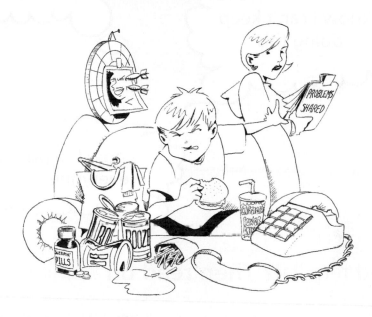

Unhelpful things we do

Helping you to help yourself
www.livinglifetothefull.com
www.fiveareas.com

Dr Nicky Dummett and Dr Chris Williams

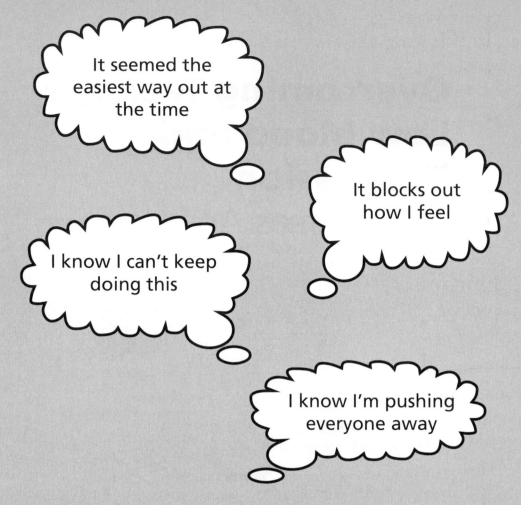

Sound familiar? **Then read on** . . .

When we have low mood or depression, it is **normal** to try to do things to feel better. This altered behaviour may be **helpful** … but sometimes it **unhelpfully messes things up**.

Often we think a behaviour is helpful when actually it's part of our problem. **Unhelpful behaviours** can make us feel better **quickly**, but later they **backfire** and make things worse for us, for example avoiding our fears, blaming other people, seeking reassurance and experimenting with drink or drugs. All these may make us feel better in the short term (which is why they can be mistaken as helpful). But in the longer term they backfire. And so they worsen how we feel physically, mentally or in our relationships.

In contrast, a truly helpful activity **stays good for us** and often for others as well.

In this workbook you will:

- Find out about how some behaviours can make things worse and backfire

- Discover key information about the vicious circle of unhelpful behaviours

- Think about other people's behaviours

- Get hints and tips to reduce unhelpful behaviours

- Make a plan to reduce any unhelpful behaviours you have been doing.

Unhelpful behaviours

Sometimes we may try to block how we feel with **unhelpful behaviours**. For example, by:

- Becoming too dependent on others

- Pushing people away

- Drinking too much alcohol or (even more worryingly) using street drugs to block how we feel (see the workbook *Alcohol, drugs and me*).

These actions often make us feel better in the short term. But they usually also backfire and create more problems in the immediate future or in the longer term. So these actions actually keep our problems from going away and become part of our problem. A **vicious circle of unhelpful behaviour** may result.

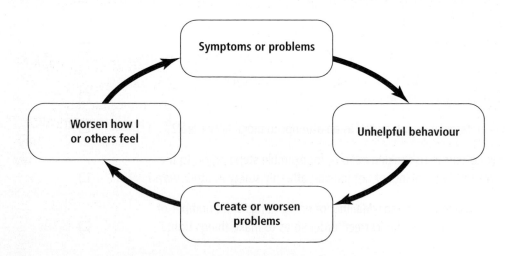

Look at the following list and tick the activity or activities you've been doing in the past few weeks. Several unhelpful behaviours have been listed here to help you to think about changes that could be happening in your own life.

As a result of how I feel, am I:	Tick here if you have noticed this – even if just sometimes
Spending a lot of time isolating myself in a 'cocoon', dwelling on things, turning them over and over in my mind?	☐
Eating too much to block how I feel ('comfort eating'), or over-eating so much that this becomes a 'binge'?	☐
Making impulsive decisions about important things, for example giving up commitments without really thinking through the consequences?	☐
Blaming others for everything?	☐
Setting myself up to fail – by setting too high standards?	☐
Trying to spend my way out of how I feel (retail therapy)?	☐
Being demanding of or always seeking reassurance from others?	☐
In place of having 'real-life' relationships around me, using television, soaps or the internet to live a fantasy life?	☐
Looking to others to make decisions or sort out problems for me?	☐
Setting myself up to be rejected by others?	☐
Throwing myself into doing things so I am so busy there are no opportunities to stop, think and reflect?	☐
Pushing others away and being verbally or physically threatening or rude to them?	☐
Deliberately harming myself in an attempt to block how I feel?	☐
Taking part in risk-taking actions, for example stepping on to the road without looking, or not looking after my safety in other ways?	☐
Compulsively checking, cleaning, or doing things a set number of times or in exactly the 'correct' order so as to make things right?	☐

Carrying out mental rituals such as counting or deliberately thinking 'good' thoughts to make things feel right? ☐

Being overly aware of and always checking for symptoms of physical illness? ☐

Relating to others in unhelpful ways, for example always giving in to others, or making excuses so as not to say what I really mean? ☐

Misusing drink or illegal drugs or even prescribed medication to block how I feel in general or improve how I sleep? ☐

Responding in other ways that aim to be a quick fix to how I feel, for example quickly leaving situations before I have the chance to settle or feel better? ☐

Write down any other unhelpful behaviours that you may have been doing here. You may also get ideas from reading the rest of the workbook.

Now ask yourself the following questions about each one of the behaviours you ticked above.

Q **Is this unhelpful in the short or longer term either for me or for other people?**

Yes ☐   No ☐   Sometimes ☐

Q **Overall has this worsened how I feel?**

Yes ☐   No ☐   Sometimes ☐

If you have answered 'Yes' or 'Sometimes' to these questions, you're going through a pattern of unhelpful behaviour.

Some examples

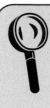

Example: Helen's vicious circle of unhelpful checking behaviour

After becoming depressed, Helen is finding it hard to concentrate. She is convinced that her brain isn't working properly. As a result she's constantly anxious about her concentration. She pays special attention to her thinking and worries she is missing important things in lessons. She even fears she may be going mad. She's always asking to check her work against Katie's, the girl who sits next to her in class, to reassure herself that she hasn't missed anything – even when she's fairly sure she hasn't. This reassurance-seeking behaviour (checking) is now really annoying Katie.

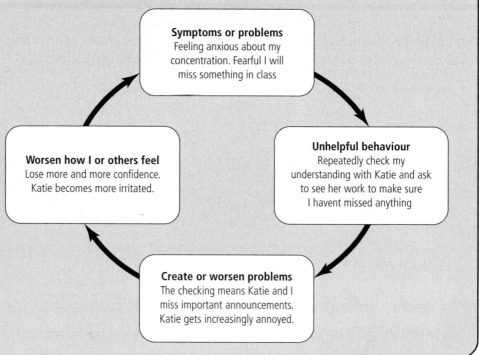

Symptoms or problems
Feeling anxious about my concentration. Fearful I will miss something in class

Unhelpful behaviour
Repeatedly check my understanding with Katie and ask to see her work to make sure I havent missed anything

Create or worsen problems
The checking means Katie and I miss important announcements. Katie gets increasingly annoyed.

Worsen how I or others feel
Lose more and more confidence. Katie becomes more irritated.

 How does Helen's constant reassurance seeking affect Helen and Katie?

Immediately

- **Physically and mentally**: whenever Helen feels anxious, checking her work against Katie's makes her **feel less tense** straight away. In the short term, she feels better.

- **Socially**: Katie is concerned to start with and wants to help.

In the longer term (over the next few weeks)

- **Physically**: Constant checking makes Helen feel more and more tired.

- **Mentally**: She feels anxious all the time about whether she has copied things correctly, loses self-confidence and feels more dependent on Katie. Her anxiety rises more and more, making it difficult for her to take in what the teacher says.

- **Socially**: Katie gets so annoyed that she stops letting Helen see her work. Finally she asks to sit with someone else, leaving Helen sitting alone in class each day.

Example: Ben's drug misuse

Ben's been out of school for many weeks and is now having worries about going back. He's also concerned whether he will ever get a job after he leaves school. He has now, very worryingly, started to experiment with street drugs to try to cope. This is affecting both him and his mum.

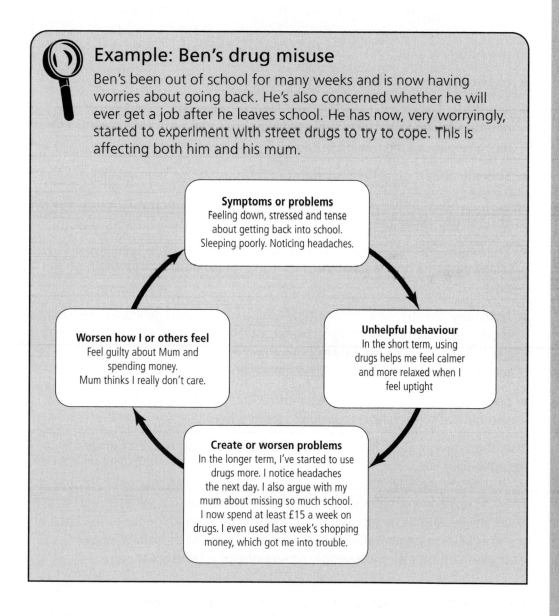

Symptoms or problems
Feeling down, stressed and tense about getting back into school. Sleeping poorly. Noticing headaches.

Unhelpful behaviour
In the short term, using drugs helps me feel calmer and more relaxed when I feel uptight

Create or worsen problems
In the longer term, I've started to use drugs more. I notice headaches the next day. I also argue with my mum about missing so much school. I now spend at least £15 a week on drugs. I even used last week's shopping money, which got me into trouble.

Worsen how I or others feel
Feel guilty about Mum and spending money.
Mum thinks I really don't care.

Ben does not think he has a drug 'problem'. Instead he sees drugs as **helpful**. This is because he hasn't worked out the **unhelpful effect** on him. He needs to start looking at the downside of misusing street drugs as well as the immediate benefits. This means looking at the short-term and longer-term effects of his daily drug use on himself and others.

Q How does Ben's drug misuse affect Ben and his mum?

Immediately

- **Physically**: Ben gets headaches and feels disconnected all day.

- **Mentally**: The drugs make Ben **feel less unhappy for a while** and help him sleep at night to begin with. But then sometimes the drugs make him feel anxious, wound up and irritable.

- **Socially**: Ben is more likely to swear at his mum when she says she is worried.

In the longer term (over a few weeks)

- **Physically**: Ben finds that he has frequent headaches, and feels sick and shaky when he hasn't used drugs for some time. He feels run down all the time.

- **Mentally**: Ben becomes increasingly anxious, angry and depressed. He spends more and more time wanting to use drugs. He notices that his mood swings are getting much worse. He feels more and more anxious than he used to. He realises he's becoming suspicious of others and even paranoid at times.

- **Socially**: Ben and his mother have more and more arguments. After shouting at a teacher he is excluded from school.

The good news is that: **if this applies to you, you can make changes** to improve your life.

Think about any examples of unhelpful behaviours you do. What effect do they have on you and those around you in the short term and longer term? Look at the checklist on pages **110–11**, and from the checklist or from your own examples choose just one example of an unhelpful behaviour.

Q What effect does this unhelpful behaviour have on me and those around me?

Immediately

● Physically:

● Mentally:

● Socially (on you and others):

In the longer term (over a few weeks):

● Physically:

● Mentally:

● Socially (on you and others):

Other people's unhelpful behaviours

When we're feeling down, having family and friends around us to offer support and a listening ear can be encouraging and helpful. But **too much help** from others can feel over the top or undermine our self-confidence. What is needed is a **balanced and supportive relationship**.

You need to give others a clear message about what you do or don't want or need (see the workbook *Being Assertive*). Try reading the *Ideas for families and friends* workbook to think about what else other people do. Remember, such changes still need to be made slowly to allow you to build confidence step by step.

Example: Is advice always helpful?

The people around us may offer 'helpful advice' all the time and want to do **everything** for us because of their concerns, friendship and love for us. Sometimes it's because they are anxious about us, or occasionally it may be because they feel guilty. Whatever the reason, when others offer too much help and want to do everything for us, their actions can backfire in several ways:

- Their 'special attention' may make us feel suffocated and frustrated. We end up feeling we're being treated like a baby. Arguments and little irritations build up.

- Although they mean well, their actions actually undermine how we feel because if others take responsibility for doing everything for us, this can damage our confidence and worsen how we feel. Another danger is that we will drop more and more of our day-to-day activities, losing things that bring us pleasure, closeness and a sense of achievement (see the *Doing things that make me feel good* workbook).

 Task

You may want to find a way to ask someone who's being over-helpful (or even bossy) to stop this behaviour – even just for a while and let you do things for yourself.

- You can start by simply letting them know the problems you have with what they do.

- Then ask them to think **together with you** about what might be better (see the workbook *Ideas for families and friends*).

- They may have been doing things because they know things you don't know. You may need to think this new information over together too.

- Sometimes it helps to brainstorm options with someone else who's less involved in your problem first of all.

Overcoming unhelpful behaviours

By working through the **seven steps** described here, you can learn how to plan clear ways to overcome unhelpful behaviours. It can be hard to do this. You may feel your unhelpful habits have gone on for so long that they're just part of your life now. You may miss the relief that they brought to you at first. So it's important **not to try to change things all at once**.

 Before you start, think: why bother with the seven steps?

You may think 'I know what I need to do – I'm just going to stop'.

You may be right – sometimes change can be down to just making one decision. But you'll find that going through the seven steps will give you a way that **you can use again and again** to tackle any kind of problem in life. The seven steps will help you plan the changes step by step so you can boost your chances of success. Even if your problems seem simple this time, we suggest you go through these seven steps and practise the approach, until it becomes second nature to you.

Step 1: Identify and define your problem as clearly as possible

Example: Ben's drug misuse

Ben has started to buy drugs from someone he knows. He realises that the drug is doing him harm. He now has mood swings and headaches, and his concentration is poor. He's also upset that he and his mum argue constantly over his drug misuse. She has surprised him by saying things have got so bad he may have to go and live with his cousins for a while if things don't improve. He decides he wants to 'do something about it'.

Ben's first task is to find out exactly how much of a problem his drug misuse is. He therefore keeps a **diary** to record his drug use in one week. (For this he uses the blank diary at the end of the workbook *Alcohol, drugs and me*.) He adds up how much he has spent every day in the week. He finds he's actually spending about £20 a week! This is a surprise for him – he had thought he was using much less than this. He thinks about all the reasons he wants to change: he'll feel better, and he wants to spend the money on some other things. He also knows it would improve things with his mother, and his mood swings are now scaring him. He therefore decides he's going to change and chooses his first target.

Ben's **target:** Ben calls the support line that he got to know about from the Talk to Frank website (www.talktofrank.com). He decides that his medium-term target over the next few weeks is **to reduce his drug use to only £5 a week, with a view to stopping altogether**.

To make these changes Ben needs to decide on a **realistic first step** to take. He decides that his first step should be to reduce his drug use to £15 a week to begin with. He knows from the Talk to Frank website that he won't get any major side effects from cutting down to £15.

- Ben's initial target: 'I want to reduce my drug use to £15 a week to begin with.'
- Ben checks: 'Is this a small, focused target I can tackle in one go?'
- He decides: 'Yes'.

He has therefore broken the problem of getting off drugs down into a **smaller first step**.

Step 2: Think of as many solutions as possible to achieve your first step

Sometimes you can find it hard to even start tackling a problem. One way around this is to try to step back and see if any other solutions are possible. This is called **brainstorming**. The more ideas you think of, the more likely it is that a good one will emerge. The idea of brainstorming is to come up with as many ideas as possible. And from among those ideas, you can find a realistic and practical solution for overcoming your problem.

Example: Ben's ideas from brainstorming

(1) I could stop drug use completely on weekdays and have all £15 at the weekend.

(2) I could plan to spread out £5 in the week and £10 at the weekend.

(3) I could plan to take the same amount each night. spreading things evenly.

(4) I could go to see the doctor or a drug clinic for help.

(5) I could give up taking drugs all in one go. I'm not going to tell anyone what I'm doing.

Step 3: Look at the pros and cons of each possible solution

Example: Ben's analysis of his possible solutions

Suggestion	Pros (advantages)	Cons (disadvantages)
(1) I could stop drug use completely on weekdays and have all £15 at the weekend	My body could recover for five days. I could still have a couple of nights out at the weekend.	I know if I have a night out in the week I'll blow it and use drugs again. I'll really have some grief then from my mum. I'd be better off not going out in the week
(2) I could plan to spread out £5 in the week and £10 at the weekend	That still adds up to £15. It would mean I wouldn't miss the drugs on any day	I'm just a bit worried if I start using more at the weekend I'll just keep wanting to keep using this amount every day

Suggestion	Pros (advantages)	Cons (disadvantages)
(3) I could plan to take the same amount each night, spreading things evenly	I like this idea. I'd spread the reduction over the whole week and it'd keep everything nice and stable. There wouldn't be any 'big' nights with far more drug use. Mum would probably like that too	It might feel quite boring. Just the same each night. It also means the weekend wouldn't be special
(4) I could go to see the doctor or a drug clinic for help	Talking to someone might encourage me to give up. It would be good to know I'm not on my own. It might give me the chance of stopping the drugs all together	I don't think I need this level of support – but I could ask for it if I found I needed it later. I want to be able to make these changes myself. I don't think I need medical support
(5) I could give up taking drugs all in one go. I'm not going to tell anyone what I'm doing	I'd feel really good to have done this in one go	I might set myself up to fail. I wish I'd never started the drugs, but I know this would feel like too big a step just now

Step 4: Choose one of the solutions

All these solutions could work. But the solution that you choose should make a sensible first step in achieving your goal. It should be **realistic** and **likely to succeed**.

Ben decides on **option 3**: I will cut my drug use to the same amount every night, spreading things evenly.

This option seems best for him. He checks it with the **questions for effective change:**

Will it be **useful** for changing how I am?

Yes, I could learn that I can start to cut it down if I use a definite plan.

Is it a **specific** task so that I will know when I have done it?

Yes, I'm clear what I am going to do – use the same amount each day. I won't even keep an extra stash in the house so I'm not tempted.

Is it something that is realistic, practical and achievable?

Yes, I could do this. It seems realistic. I know from the helpline that if I cut this much I should be OK whereas if I tried to stop all at once I'd probably not succeed as I might have withdrawal symptoms – I wouldn't want that.

Step 5: Plan the steps needed to carry out your chosen solution

Ben's plan: I'll split the week's supply into seven and set it out in my room. That way, if I'm tempted to use more any day I can see it means less for the next day. This will be the only supply I let myself buy.

He then goes through the rest of the **questions for effective change**.

 Does it make clear exactly **what** I am going to do and **when** I am going to do it?

Yes, I know what I'm going to do and I'll start tomorrow.

Is it an activity that won't be easily blocked by practical problems?

What could prevent this? I'm due to go to Bob's party next Saturday. There's bound to be people using drugs there – I'll just take the day's supply with me and no more. I'll steer clear of getting any more by not taking any money with me.

Will I learn useful things even if it doesn't work out perfectly?

Yes.

Ben has answered 'Yes' to each of the questions. If he hadn't, he would have needed to think what changes he could make to change or improve his plan.

Key point

Planning should include how you will react if things don't work out.

Ben builds in some thought on this: *If I mess up and end up taking too much any day, I'll still carry on with the plan and continue with it the next day rather than giving up.*

Step 6: Carry out the plan

Example: Ben carries out his plan

Ben manages to put his plan into action for the first few days and feels quite good about himself and how things are going. But things don't go according to plan when he goes to Bob's party. He uses his own supply that he brought with him, and then thinks 'What the heck, let your hair down'. He ends up borrowing money, has to walk five miles home and has a blazing row with his mum. The next day he wakes up feeling worse and thinks 'I'm obviously not strong enough to do this. Maybe I should just give up completely'.

After a few hours, however, he remembers he'd thought that there would be occasional hiccups. And that he'd planned to go ahead with his solution if things went wrong. He realises, 'If I just get back to my plan every time things go wrong, things have to work out OK. The only way they won't is if I give up'.

Ben can also learn from what happened and plan to avoid making the same mistake again: social situations like parties mean he is more likely to overdo things. He doesn't want to stop going to parties but he needs to plan better ways of coping – for example by telling people at the start that he doesn't want any more than a certain amount.

Ben therefore starts to go along with his plan again the next day and uses just his daily limit for the rest of the week. By the end of the week he finds he feels more confident about his ability to handle things next time he goes to a party.

Step 7: Review your learning

> ### Example: Ben's review
> Was my selected approach successful?
>
> Yes ☑   No ☐
>
> *Things have gone quite well. I managed to get down to £15 in total over the second week. There was that problem at Bob's party, but I've managed to move on. Just because a set-back occurs does not mean that everything is over.*
>
> Did it help me to tackle my target problem?
>
> Yes ☑   No ☐
>
> Did I have any problems using this approach?
>
> Yes ☑   No ☐
>
> What have I learned from doing this?
>
> *Try to stick to the plan if things go wrong. Don't give up, but try to adjust so that I get back on target. Others can really help – Mum's been fantastic. We also now seem to be getting on a lot better. I've really valued her support.*

Now try it out yourself

We've shown you how Ben could use the **seven-step approach** for his problem. But you can use it to change **any** unhelpful behaviour.

Apply what you have learned from Ben's example, and use the questions below to help **you** to work through the seven-step approach to reduce your own unhelpful behaviour.

Step 1: Identify and define your problem as clearly as possible

It isn't possible to deal with every problem all at once. First go back to the checklist of unhelpful behaviours you completed (page **110**). Choose **one** unhelpful behaviour you want to tackle. If people try to change everything at once there's a big chance that they might fail. So if you've ticked many boxes in the checklist, **choose the unhelpful behaviour that you wish to change first.**

Task

Write down your chosen problem here.

To begin with, keep a record your unhelpful behaviour over several days. A diary may be the best way (for example the one at the back of this workbook, on page **136**). Make a note of:

- When the behaviour or thing you've been doing occurs
- How much and how often in a typical day or week you do this behaviour or activity (for example how many times you've sought reassurance, how much money you've spent)
- How long it lasts for.

This information will help you to clearly identify the unhelpful behaviour that needs to be changed. It will give you an idea of how much it is happening and how big a job it will be to change. You can read the example about Ben if you need help or you can discuss it with someone you trust.

Now ask yourself if you need to break down tackling this problem area into smaller, more achievable, steps. If you think so, write your first step here:

Check again: Is this a small focused problem I can realistically tackle in one step?

Yes ☐   Go to the next step

No ☐   Break it down again until you answer 'Yes'.

Step 2: Think of as many solutions as possible to achieve your first step

Try to **think broadly**. Here are some useful questions for thinking up possible solutions.

- What advice would you give a friend who was trying to tackle the same problem? It's often easier to think of solutions for others than for ourselves.
- What **ridiculous** solutions can I include as well as more sensible ones?
- What helpful ideas would others (for example family or friends) suggest?
- What approaches have I tried in the past in similar circumstances?

If you feel stuck, brainstorming with someone you trust can be helpful.

Brainstorming my problem
My ideas (including ridiculous ones) are:

1

2

3

4

5

Step 3: Look at the pros and cons of each possible solution

My suggestion	Pros (advantages)	Cons (disadvantages)

Step 4: Choose one of the solutions

Bear in mind the pros and cons you've come up with and choose one solution.

Remember, the solution you're looking for as a first step is something that gets you moving in the right direction – small enough to be possible over the next week, but big enough to move you forwards.

Write down your chosen solution here.

Next, check it with the **questions for effective change:**

Q Will it be **useful** for changing how I am?

Yes ☐ No ☐

Is it a **specific** task so that I will know when I have done it?

Yes ☐ No ☐

It is something that is realistic, practical and achievable.

Yes ☐ No ☐

Step 5: Plan the steps needed to carry out your chosen solution

Write down the practical steps needed to carry out your plan so that you know exactly **what** you are going to do, and **when** you are going to do it. Include ways of tackling any blocks that might get in the way.

My plan to reduce my unhelpful behaviour:

Now check your plan with the rest of the **questions for effective change**:

 Does it make clear exactly **what** I am going to do and **when** I am going to do it?

Yes ☐   No ☐

Is it an activity that won't be easily blocked by practical problems?

Yes ☐   No ☐

Will I learn useful things even if it doesn't work out perfectly?

Yes ☐   No ☐

You should have answered 'Yes' to each of the questions. If you haven't, try to change things until you can answer 'Yes' to all the questions.

Key point

Remember, you can achieve large changes by moving one step at a time. Don't push yourself too hard because that can backfire.

Your plan must include how you will react if things don't work out. Write down your plan of what to do if things don't work out here.

Step 6: Carry out your plan
Good luck!

Step 7: Review your learning
Write down what happened here.

Q Was my selected approach successful?

Yes ☐   No ☐

Did it help me tackle my chosen problem?

Yes ☐   No ☐

Did I have any problems using this approach?

Yes ☐   No ☐

What have I learnt from doing this?
Write down any helpful lessons or information you have learned from what happened. If things didn't go quite as you hoped, try to learn from this.

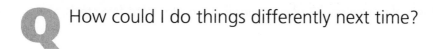 How could I do things differently next time?

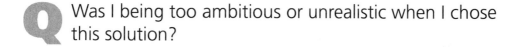 Was I being too ambitious or unrealistic when I chose this solution?

Planning the next steps

 Example: Ben's next steps

Ben has cut his drug use to £15 a week.

- His **medium-term** target is to reduce his drug use to £5 over the next two weeks.

- His **long-term** target is to be off drugs completely.

He needs to have a clear step-by-step plan that is likely to be successful. He therefore needs to plan sensible changes for the next steps to take him where he wants to go.

Ben's next steps	Time
Using £15 over the week	During this week (week 1)
Using £15 over the week	During week 2
Using £10 over the week	During week 3
Using £5 over the week	During week 4
Not using at all	After that

Ben's longer-term plan to stop drugs completely is made up of five steps.

> ## Key point
>
> Each of Ben's steps can be planned out in detail using the same seven-step approach. Each one builds on the previous ones to help to move forwards. Over many weeks this can add up to a **big overall change**.

Your plan

Now that you've looked at how your first planned step went, the next step is to plan another change to build on this.

You have the choice to:

- Stick at the target you have achieved
- Focus on the same unhelpful behaviour but plan to reduce it further
- Select a new unhelpful behaviour to work on.

Think about the pros and cons of each of these choices.

Choosing the next unhelpful behaviour to reduce

The key is to **use the seven steps again** to create your own clear plan.

Do

- Plan to alter **only one** unhelpful behaviour over any one week.
- Make an **action plan** to slowly alter what you do in an effective and planned way.
- Ask yourself the **questions for effective change** to check that your plan should work.
- **Write down** your action plan in detail so that you're clear about what you will be doing.

Don't

- Try to change too many things all at once.
- Choose something that is too big a target to start with.
- Be negative and think, 'Nothing can be done, what's the point, it's a waste of time'. Instead, try to experiment to find out if this negative thinking is really helpful.

Write your **longer-term plan** here.

- What I will do over the next week:

- What I will do over the week after that:

- What I will do over the week after that:

- What I hope to be doing one month from now:

- What I hope to be doing six months from now:

- What I hope to be doing one year from now:

Remember: plan **what** you will do and **when** you will do it. **Learn** from what happens so that you can keep putting what you have learned into practice. By doing this, you will be able to bring about slow but steady changes in a planned, step-by-step way. In this way, you will slowly rebuild your confidence and increase your control over any unhelpful behaviours.

Summary

In this workbook you have:

- Learnt about unhelpful ways of responding to problems

- Learnt about the vicious circle of unhelpful behaviours

- Discovered some tips about ways to reduce unhelpful behaviours

- Practised a step-by-step approach to plan how you will reduce an unhelpful behaviour.

Let's look at the whole picture again

After you've been putting this workbook into action in your life for a while, rate the size of your problems again in each of the **five areas**.

Q Overall, do I have (or have I had) problems in Area 1: People and events?

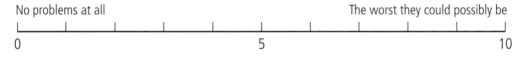

No problems at all   The worst they could possibly be

0   5   10

Q Overall, do I have problems in Area 2: Altered thinking?

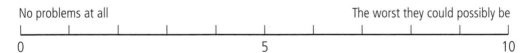

No problems at all   The worst they could possibly be

0   5   10

Q Overall, do I have problems in Area 3: Altered feelings?

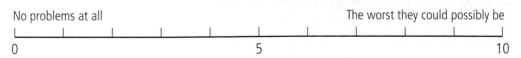

No problems at all   The worst they could possibly be

0   5   10

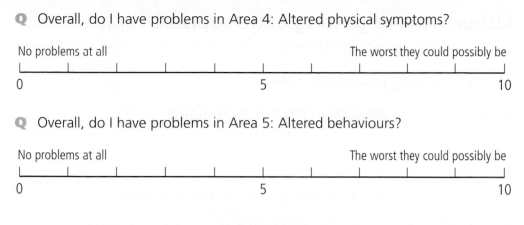

Q Overall, do I have problems in Area 4: Altered physical symptoms?

No problems at all   The worst they could possibly be

0   5   10

Q Overall, do I have problems in Area 5: Altered behaviours?

No problems at all   The worst they could possibly be

0   5   10

Q What have I learnt from this review?

Q What do I want to try next?

Putting into practice what you have learnt

Try to continue to put into practice what you have learnt over the next few weeks. Don't try to solve every problem you face all at once. Plan out what to do at a pace that is right for you. Build changes one step at a time.

Other ways of getting extra support

Think about how to get support from:

- Your general practitioner (GP)
- Other healthcare practitioners you have worked with
- Friends you can trust
- Your family
- Websites – for example Talk to Frank (www.talktofrank.com)
- **Yourself** – because ultimately it's down to you to plan to change.

Other ways of getting more information and support:

- Read the section 'Sources of extra help' in the *Understanding why I feel as I do* workbook.

 Do the on-line module at **www.livinglifetothefull.com** or use the support forum there to swap ideas and encouragement. Find extra self-help resources and ideas at **www.fiveareas.com**.

A request for feedback

The content of this workbook is updated and improved on a regular basis based on feedback from readers and practitioners. If there are areas in the workbook that you found hard to understand or that seemed unclear, please let us know. However, we don't provide any specific advice on treatment.

To provide feedback please contact us:

 Via our website forum: **www.livinglifetothefull.com**

Or by e-mail: **feedback@fiveareas.com**. In your feedback, please can you state which workbook or book you are referring to.

My notes

My unhelpful behaviour diary

Day and date	Morning	Afternoon	Evening	Add up the total time (or money) spent
Monday				Total =
Tuesday				Total =
Wednesday				Total =
Thursday				Total =
Friday				Total =
Saturday				Total =
Sunday				Total =

Remember to record **every** time you do the unhelpful behaviour

Week's total =

Overcoming Teenage Low Mood and Depression

A Five Areas Approach

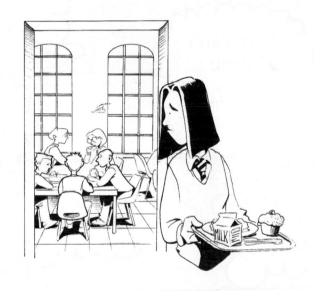

Restarting things we've avoided

Helping you to help yourself
www.livinglifetothefull.com
www.fiveareas.com

Dr Nicky Dummett and Dr Chris Williams

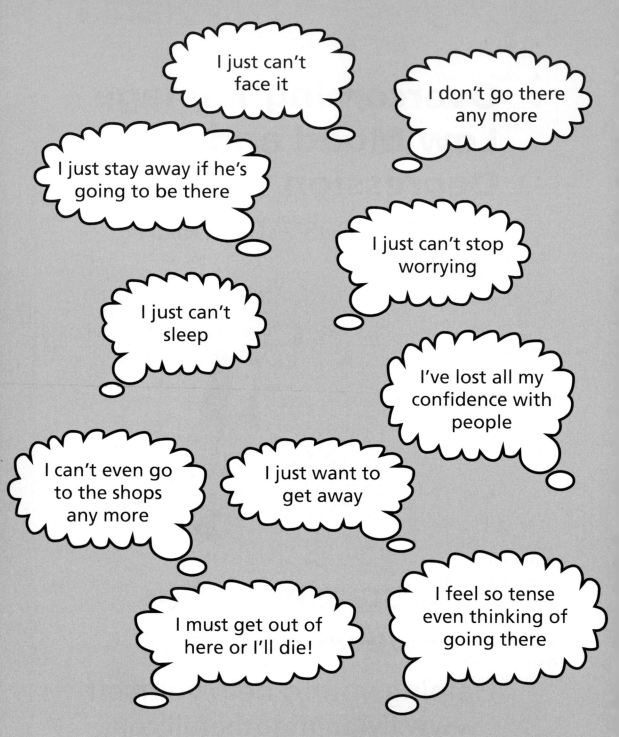

... is this you?

If it is ... this **workbook is for you**.

Overcoming Teenage Low Mood and Depression: A Five Areas Approach

In this workbook you will:

- Learn how avoiding and escaping from things affects our life

- Learn to identify any avoidance in your own life and think about its effect on you

- Read an example of how to overcome avoidance

- Learn how to make slow, steady changes to your life and also some next steps to build on this improvement.

When we feel low we often start to worry about what we can do and what we can't do. We may begin to **avoid doing** or **escape** (exit) from things. We try to avoid:

- **Particular people, places or situations where we think we will feel worse**. For example, people who feel panicky in crowded areas (this is sometimes called agoraphobia) will avoid going into larger, busier shops.

- **Communication**. For example, someone who feels very anxious when talking to people will avoid conversations they need to have.

But ...

Avoidance and escaping make things worse because:

- We don't see that what we are scared of usually doesn't actually happen

- They wrongly teach us that the **only** way to deal with a difficult situation is to avoid or escape from it

- We lose contact with people and don't sort out misunderstandings.

So a **vicious circle of avoidance** often results and we avoid and escape more and more. This worsens our anxiety and saps our confidence. We stop doing more and more things so our lives get really restricted. We also lose touch with people.

Example: Helen's anxieties

Helen is worried whenever she goes to the lunch hall that friends she has fallen out with will be there. She says 'I'm not going to the lunch hall if they might be there because I'll get panicky. I'd really feel hot and sweaty and start breathing very fast. I'd be scared they'd laugh at me and think I look stupid. Instead, I'll even miss lunch if I have to.' Because of her fears Helen is avoiding things. This is undermining her confidence and adding to her problems.

Are you avoiding or escaping?

To see if you're avoiding or escaping from problems or situations, ask yourself:

- What have I stopped or **avoided** doing because of my worries or concerns?
- What have I started to leave or **escape** from because of my worries or concerns?

  *Remember that at times your way of avoiding things can be quite **subtle**, for example you may choose to miss important things because it's scary meeting people.*

Write your answers here.

I am avoiding:

I often escape from:

Now reflect on your answers using the following three questions.

Q Am I avoiding things or escaping from doing things because of feeling anxious?

Yes ☐   No ☐   Sometimes ☐

Q Has this reduced my confidence in things and led to an increasingly restricted life?

Yes ☐   No ☐   Sometimes ☐

Q Overall has this worsened how I feel?

Yes ☐   No ☐   Sometimes ☐

If you have answered 'Yes' or 'Sometimes' to all three questions, then you are going through a vicious circle of avoidance.

But there's some good news

One really good way of tackling our fears is to face up to them **in a planned step-by-step way**. Once you have noticed that you're avoiding or escaping from things, you can begin to start working on tackling this. You will find out how to do this in this workbook.

Similarly, if we communicate well then we let other people know what we're thinking and feeling. We also find out what they are thinking and feeling so we can understand each other better and solve problems and misunderstandings together. The *Being assertive* workbook will help you do this.

Why escaping doesn't help ... but facing up to fears does help

As you will read in the last section of this workbook, a really good way of tackling our fears is to face up to them. This is because if we stay in a situation that we are scared of, **eventually the fear wears out and goes away**. Scientists have shown that this is because the chemicals that send fear messages to our brain eventually literally run out. That's why facing up to fears works. Slowly, by facing up to fear, we can overcome it.

To start with, it can take 5 or 20 minutes or even an hour or longer for fear to go away, depending on how scared we've been **if we stay with it long enough to feel better**. Also, next time we face the same situation we don't get so scared because we've learnt that the fear will go if we face it.

Overcoming Teenage Low Mood and Depression: A Five Areas Approach   © Dr Nicky Dummet and Dr Chris Williams (2008)

*The best way to face up to fears is to do it **one step at a time**. This means breaking our plan to tackle the fear into steps so that each step is never too big, too scary or too overwhelming.*

So, to face up to any fear we need to:

- Break things down into small steps, so that each step is something we can manage **without too much difficulty** and **without having to escape**.

- Allow **enough time** for us to stay until the fear has reduced and to not escape before then. If we escape **before we have started to feel better**, we don't see that the fear wears out. And we're also much more likely to escape next time because we have just practised escaping again.

- Make sure you repeat each step a few times before moving on to the next step. This will build your confidence more and more.

Example: How staying in a situation that makes us anxious can be helpful

If we do or think something that makes us feel anxious (but not overwhelmed by fear) and stay with it, our fear might do something like **Line 1** in the figure below. But if we stay with the situation until we feel better, we find that the next time we are in the situation our fear isn't so bad (**Line 2**) and the time after that it's even less (**Line 3**), and so on. So, for each step of our recovery we need to make ourselves face our fear and stay with it several times to reduce our fear, build our confidence and make moving on to the next step easier.

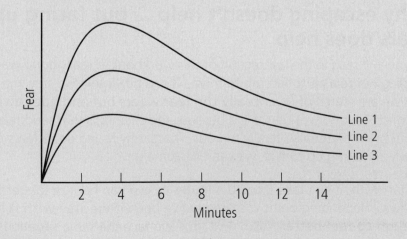

What do I want to tackle first?

The most important thing about moving forwards is selecting which changes to try to make first. By choosing one or a few activities to start with, you're actively choosing at first **not** to focus on other areas. The following checklist will help you get started.

As a result of feeling anxious or worried, am I:	Tick here if you have noticed this – even if just sometimes
Avoiding certain situations, objects, places or people?	☐
Avoiding dealing with important practical problems (both large and small)?	☐
Not really being honest with others? For example, saying yes when I really mean no or by not saying things that I really want to	☐
Trying hard to avoid situations that trigger upsetting thoughts or memories?	☐
Avoiding physical activity or exercise that I should be doing for my physical health?	☐
Avoiding opening or replying to letters, e-mails or texts?	☐
Sleeping in to avoid doing things or meeting people?	☐
Looking to others to sort things out for me?	☐
Avoiding answering the phone or the door when people visit?	☐
Avoiding talking to other people face to face?	☐
Avoiding being with others in crowded or hot places, or avoiding busy or large shops?	☐
Avoiding going on buses, in cars, in taxis etc., or to any places where it's hard to escape?	☐
Avoiding walking alone away from home?	☐
No longer attending activities or clubs because it feels just too much to cope with at present?	☐
Avoiding anything else?	☐

Now look at what you've ticked and choose **one** target area to focus on first. If you've ticked many boxes in the checklist, bear in mind you'll find it hard to overcome all these areas at once. Instead you need to decide which one area you're going to start with.

My target activity

Remember that this should be something you have avoided, and not doing it has worsened how you feel.

*The key to starting to do your chosen activity again is to use a **step-by-step** approach. You break down the activity into small steps so that no step seems too large. In this way you plan a **steady and slow increase** in your activity to help tackle your problems and rebuild your confidence.*

Your first step

Your first step needs to get you moving in the right direction. It should be something you can realistically manage in the next week or two. For example, if your target activity is to feel comfortable in shops again, think of the most fear you have ever felt doing this and rate that as 100 per cent fear level (so 0 per cent would be having no fear). Try to think of ways to face your fear that you think will give you around 20 per cent or 30 per cent of your fear – **whatever is realistic for you as a first step**. For example, if you're afraid to got to a shop alone, go in with someone you trust or just stand outside the first time, whatever you think will be 20–30 per cent scary, and stay there until you feel better.

 ## Example: Helen's avoidance

Helen decides to sit with **anyone** where there's a space at lunch, rather than try to only sit with friends or other people from her year. She thinks this will be about 25 per cent scary.

Key point

Your first step should be something that helps you tackle your avoidance. It should be a bit scary but not so scary that you can't do it. You must be realistic in your choice so that your target doesn't seem impossible, and you won't end up having to escape.

Q Ask yourself, is this first step:

- Realistic and achievable so that I'm likely to succeed?

  Yes ☐   No ☐

- Not so scary that I can't face doing it?

  Yes ☐   No ☐

- Still big enough to move me forward?

  Yes ☐   No ☐

My first step will be:

Now see if you can answer 'Yes' to the three questions below about your chosen step:

Q Will it be **useful** for changing how you are?

Yes ☐   No ☐

Is it a **specific** task so that you'll know when you've done it?

Yes ☐   No ☐

Is it something that is realistic, practical and achievable?

Yes ☐   No ☐

If you answered 'Yes' to all three questions your chosen step should help start you off. If not, please go back and choose another target.

Plan the steps needed to carry it out

*You need to make a clear **overall plan** that will help you decide exactly what steps you're going to do to build up to where you want to be. Your plan should also say roughly when you will do them. Consider how long it will take and think of possible problems that might arise. Remember to build into your plan some thought about what you'll do if the plan doesn't fully succeed.*

It's useful to write down each of the steps that you'll need for your plan.

The steps in my overall plan

Making a clear plan is the important part of your problem-solving process. Be as clear as possible in your plan. Write here exactly **how** you're going do the first step of your plan and **when** you're going to do it (include ways of tackling any possible blocks that might get in the way).

How and **when** I will do the first step of my plan:

What if a step doesn't work out? Write your plan of what you can do next here.

Ask yourself the **questions for effective change**.

Q Is this step one that:

- Will be **useful** for understanding or changing how I am?

  Yes ☐   No ☐

- Is a **specific** task so that I'll know when I have done it?

  Yes ☐   No ☐

- Is realistic, practical and achievable?

  Yes ☐   No ☐

- Makes clear what I am going to do and when I am going to do it?

  Yes ☐   No ☐

- Is an activity that won't be easily blocked or prevented by practical problems?

  Yes ☐   No ☐

- Will help me to learn useful things even if it doesn't work out perfectly?

  Yes ☐   No ☐

You should be able to answer 'Yes' to each question.

And once again: remember to build into your plan what you'll do if the plan doesn't fully succeed.

What I will do if this step doesn't fully succeed:

Example: Helen uses the questions for effective change to help review her plan

Q Will it be useful for understanding or changing how I am?

At the moment, I always try to eat at quieter times like just before the canteen shuts, and then rush my food. If I could change that rushing in and out at the end and be able to eat whenever it's convenient for me, that would be a very useful first step. I also always feel I have to try to sit with my age group. I can usually chat with younger people without a problem, but I do need to build my confidence with people my own age again. If I practise sitting with younger as well as older people, I may learn that I don't always have to sit with people my age or always have 'friends' to sit with to feel OK about myself. This may then be a useful first step in building my confidence generally.

I know from other times I've been scared of things that the fear usually goes away after a while if you just face the problem and stay in the situation. I'd like to give myself the chance to see if this can happen with this problem if I can face it and stay in the situation.

Q Is it a specific task so that I will know when I have done it?

I need to be clear about what I'm going to do. I will go into the canteen when it's convenient for me and at least 40 minutes before it shuts. It doesn't matter who I sit next to, as long as I go and sit next to someone. Instead of rushing to eat my food, I will try to eat it at a normal speed until I have finished it. I don't have to try to start a conversation, but I will join in if it happens naturally.

Q Is it realistic, practical and achievable?

Is it realistic? Yes, I can do that. It's really only a little bit scary (25 per cent). I'm sure I can do this.

Q Does it make clear what I am going to do and when I am going to do it?

I have a clear idea of what I need to do. I will move around and eat in the canteen in a relaxed way and spend at least 40 minutes there. I need to think about how I can spend the extra time there. I could read the menu board, or look at the salad selection. Even better, I could give myself the time to ask for better descriptions of the food at the service area. That's something that could take a few minutes. I need to decide when I am going to do this. I think I should do it tomorrow.

Q Is it an activity that won't be easily blocked or prevented by practical problems?

Now then, what might block it? If there are lots of people from my year, I might worry people will think it's odd that I'm not sitting with them. I could plan to go at the busiest time, when we all know there's so little space all the years end up muddled together anyway. The only other thing that I can predict could stop me doing this is if I lose my nerve, and I try to start rushing round when I get there. If I have that temptation, I just need to make sure I slow down my breathing, and also my walking and eating. I'll deliberately try to just slow down, maybe concentrate on my breathing and stay in the situation at least for a few more minutes before moving on. I know from before that I'm going to notice my usual fear that 'I will do or say something stupid in front of people'. I need to be aware of that and try to challenge this fear.

Q Will it help me to learn useful things even if it doesn't work out perfectly?

I'm pretty sure this will all be okay. But if it is too scary and I really can't cope, then I'll think again and pick something less scary instead from the other options on my list. I do think I can do this though and even if it does go wrong, I'm sure I'll have learnt something.

And now … just do it!

 Task

Your task is to carry out the first step of your plan (for example during the next week). Write down exactly when you will do it so it's clear when you will put it into practice. Carry out the plan and see how it goes.

 Key point

Remember that as you do your chosen step you're undermining your old doubts and fears by **acting against them**. Pay attention to the thoughts you have before, during and afterwards about what will happen.

My review

Q How did it go?

Q Did I find the approach helpful?

Yes ☐   No ☐

Q Did it help improve things for me?

Yes ☐   No ☐

Q Did I have any problems while making these changes?

Yes ☐   No ☐

Q What have I learnt from doing this?

Q What is my next step going to be?

Learning from my review

If things didn't go quite as you hoped, write here any helpful lessons or information you have learned. Choosing realistic targets for change is important.

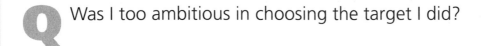 **Was I too ambitious in choosing the target I did?**

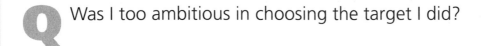 **Did something unexpected happen, for example something didn't happen as planned, or someone reacted in an unexpected way?**

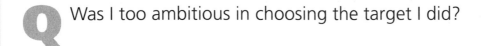 **How could I make things different next time I tackle the problem?**

 Example: How does Helen's plan go?

Helen goes into the canteen the next day when it's busy. Before she enters the canteen, she notes her anxious thoughts but reminds herself that if she carries out the plan this will help give up the old fears. She notes one fear in particular: 'If I talk to anyone, I will end up saying or doing something that gives the impression there must be something wrong with me.' She challenges it by reminding herself that even in recent weeks when she has spoken to people elsewhere, this hasn't happened. When she's got her food, she ends up on a table with three other people already there. They are two younger girls and a school prefect. Her belief that they will think she's strange because she hasn't got friends to sit with shoots up and she feels very anxious.

She thinks about leaving and begins to feel hot and sweaty, and notices an increase in her heart rate and her breathing. She starts to pile food on to her fork to try to get her meal finished and out of the situation as quickly as possible. But then she remembers that she had decided that if she felt like this she would try to control her breathing and slow down her eating. Helen makes a big effort and puts down her fork and asks the prefect to pass the water. He passes the water to her, and she pours herself a drink and realises this is the first time in ages she has even thought to get some water at lunchtime. She takes a sip between mouthfuls and chews slowly. She does this for a couple of minutes and begins to feel much better. She even notices what the food tastes like for a change.

Helen's anxiety and belief that she will say or do something to make herself look like there's something wrong with her slowly drop. She finishes eating at a normal pace and is pleasantly surprised when one of the younger girls asks her advice about where to put some food she is embarrassed that she can't finish. They talk and even end up having a laugh about it, with the girl feeling much less worried before they part. When Helen leaves, she is surprised to find that she was in the canteen for almost 45 minutes. Her belief in her fear and her feelings of anxiety have nearly gone.

Example: Helen's review.

That went really well! I hadn't expected it to.

I was almost thrown when there were only four of us at the table and no one else joined us. That hardly ever happens. I thought it'd make it much more obvious that I had no friends to sit with and also how anxious I was feeling. I was also worried that if I spoke everyone would hear if I said anything I'd regret.

Helen thinks about what she has learnt:

- Just how useful it is to have predicted what to do if I began to feel worse. When that happened I felt really scared. I remembered that I had planned to slow down my breathing and my eating if that happened. It worked! I felt a lot better – especially after slowing my eating with sips of water.

- All my concerns about them thinking I had something wrong with me because I had no friends to sit with just weren't true. It hadn't even occurred to them to think that. What's more they even thought I looked like someone they could ask for advice!

- The anxiety and physical symptoms didn't continue to rise and what's more they did gradually go away. This is such a relief. I must also say I even feel a bit proud of myself for sticking with it and learning these things!

By doing the same thing every lunchtime over the next week, Helen's anxiety becomes less and less intense. It also lasts for shorter and shorter lengths of time. By repeatedly facing her fears she is able to challenge her fearful thoughts as well as tackling her anxious feelings.

This same pattern happens no matter which fear is being tackled. Facing up to a fear causes it to slowly lose its hold on you.

Key point

By facing up to your fears in a planned way you can overcome them.

Planning the next steps

Do

- Continue to plan to change only **one** area of avoidance at a time.

- Break down the problem into **smaller parts** that each build towards your eventual goal. There can be as many or as few steps as you want in your plan.

- Produce a plan to slowly change what you do in an effective way.

- Be **realistic** in your goals.

- Use the **questions for effective change** to help plan each step.

- Write down your plan in detail so that you'll be able to put it into practice this week.

- If you find any step too hard, **go back a stage and regain your confidence**. Then, decide on another next step that's not quite so hard. Repeat this step successfully several times before trying again with the step you found too difficult.

Don't

- Choose something that is too big a target to do next.

- Try to start to change too many areas of your life all at once.

- Be negative and think 'Nothing can be done'. Instead, try to experiment to find out if this negative thinking is true or helpful.

- Try to move too quickly from one step to the next. Instead, make sure you repeatedly succeed at each step first.

You can deal with most problems in this way. Remember, the commonest reason for a plan not to work is if you are **too ambitious** or allow yourself to believe that change is impossible.

Hints and tips for tackling avoidance

- Use what you have learned earlier to write your action plan.

- Plan **what** you will do and **when** you will do it.

- Learn from what happens so that you can keep putting what you have learnt into practice.

- By doing this, you will be able to slowly rebuild your confidence, and increase your feelings of pleasure and achievement.

My next target is:

Making a weekly action plan

Each week you can build these targets one upon another. This will move you forwards one step at a time.

Example: Helen's weekly plan

Helen plans out the different steps that she needs to complete over the next few weeks. Her plan should also include reducing and stopping doing some of the more subtle types of avoidance she has noticed like avoiding making any eye contact with people of her own age.

Note that her fear rating of her first step of sitting with anyone has already gone from 25 per cent to around just 5 per cent most days. She has ticked this as completed in her plan below.

Helen's weekly targets	Expected fear level at first (0–100 per cent)	Time scale
1. Going into the canteen, sitting next to anyone (can be anyone) and staying there even if it feels uncomfortable for at least 40 minutes	Hardly scary at all 5–10 per cent scary	Week 1 as long as it's repeated at least twice ✓
2. As above, but make eye contact and smile at someone my age across the canteen at least once each lunchtime	A little scary 15 per cent scary	Week 2 Repeat at least twice
3. As above, but do it when they are closer to me and just say a casual hello	Quite scary 35 per cent scary	Week 3 and then repeat at least twice
4. As above, but try to sit near (same table) to people my age (can be anyone) each time I go in	Pretty scary 50 per cent scary at first	Weeks 4 and 5 and then repeat at least twice

Helen's weekly targets	Expected fear level (0–100 per cent)	Time scale
5. As above, but sit right next to people my age (can be anyone) each time I go in	Moderately scary 75 per cent scary	Week 6 and then repeat at least twice
6. As above, but sit near (same table) to Debbie and my other former close friends who seem to have rejected me in recent months	Very scary 85 per cent scary	Week 7 and then repeat at least twice
7. Ultimate target. To be able to go into the canteen to eat at any time and feel comfortable whomever I sit next to (including Debbie and other people I've felt rejected by)	Very scary 90 per cent now (but it used to be 100 per cent)	Week 8 and then repeat at least twice

You can see that Helen's plan is made up of many separate targets. Each next target on the way can be planned out in detail. Each new target builds upon the previous one to help Helen to move forwards.

Helen's plan helps her to face up to her fear in a planned and paced way. This means that she never feels so anxious that she wants to give up. By repeating each new stage several times each week, she can build up her confidence before moving on to the next step. If she found that a particular stage is too difficult, she could always take a step back, and replan the task.

By succeeding in these planned steady steps, real progress can be achieved. What's more, as Helen manages her fear at each target level, she finds that the next target becomes less fearful as she approaches it too.

Overcoming Teenage Low Mood and Depression: A Five Areas Approach © Dr Nicky Dummet and Dr Chris Williams (2008)

Task

Write down the next few weeks of your step-by-step approach:

My step-by-step targets	Initial fear or scariness level (0–100 per cent)	Time scale (weeks)

But remember – small steps at a time!

The key is to do everything at the right pace, so that change happens. Slow sure steps forward are the best way to make progress.

Some practical hints and tips if communication is something we have avoided

- Be realistic about your timing if you are planning to discuss an important subject. Don't surprise someone with it. For example, if you want to discuss something with a busy parent who works, don't choose the time right after they've struggled through traffic to get home after a long day at work. Try to find a better time.

- It may be that you and your relative or friend just haven't had enough positive (enjoyable) time together in general recently. Try to find some things that you enjoy doing together so you can each be reminded of the friendly, supportive side of the other.

- You may need to build up your skills bit by bit by trying to have more open communication about simple everyday things before you move on to more difficult discussions.

Don't worry that you have to make big changes in one go. Are there any small things you can try doing differently as an experiment to see whether anything can start to help?

Putting into practice what you have learnt

Carry out a series of **action plans** over the next few weeks to tackle your avoidance. If you have problems, just do what you can.

Summary

In this workbook you have:

- Learnt how avoidance and escape affect our lives

- Identified any avoidance or escaping in your own life and thought about its effect on you

- Read an example of how to overcome avoidance

- Learnt about how to plan to make slow, steady changes to your life, and also some next steps to build on this improvement.

Let's look at the whole picture again

After you have been putting this workbook into action in your life for a while, rate the size of your problems again in each of the **five areas**.

Q Overall, do I have (or have I had) problems in Area 1: People and events?

No problems at all   The worst they could possibly be

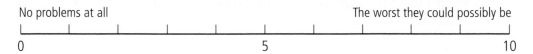

0   5   10

Q Overall, do I have problems in Area 2: Altered thinking?

No problems at all   The worst they could possibly be

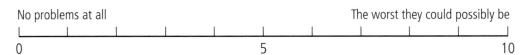

0   5   10

Q Overall, do I have problems in Area 3: Altered feelings?

No problems at all   The worst they could possibly be

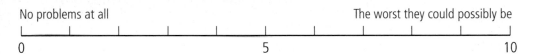

0   5   10

Q Overall, do I have problems in Area 4: Altered physical symptoms?

No problems at all   The worst they could possibly be

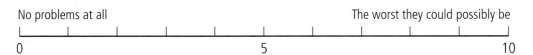

0   5   10

Q Overall, do I have problems in Area 5: Altered behaviours?

No problems at all   The worst they could possibly be

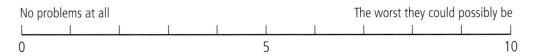

0   5   10

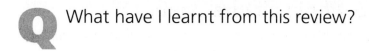

Q What have I learnt from this review?

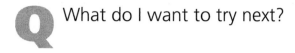

Q What do I want to try next?

A request for feedback

The content of this workbook is updated and improved on a regular basis based on feedback from readers and practitioners. If there are areas in the workbook that you found hard to understand or that seemed unclear, please let us know. However, we don't provide any specific advice on treatment.

To provide feedback please contact us:

 Via our website forum: **www.livinglifetothefull.com**

Or by e-mail: **feedback@fiveareas.com**. In your feedback, please can you state which workbook or book you are referring to.

My notes

Overcoming Teenage Low Mood and Depression

A Five Areas Approach

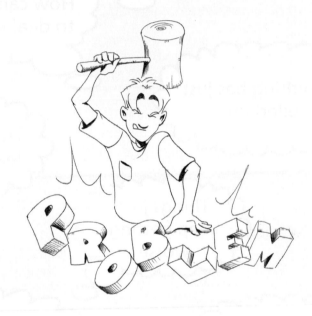

Practical problem solving

Helping you to help yourself
www.livinglifetothefull.com
www.fiveareas.com

Dr Nicky Dummett and Dr Chris Williams

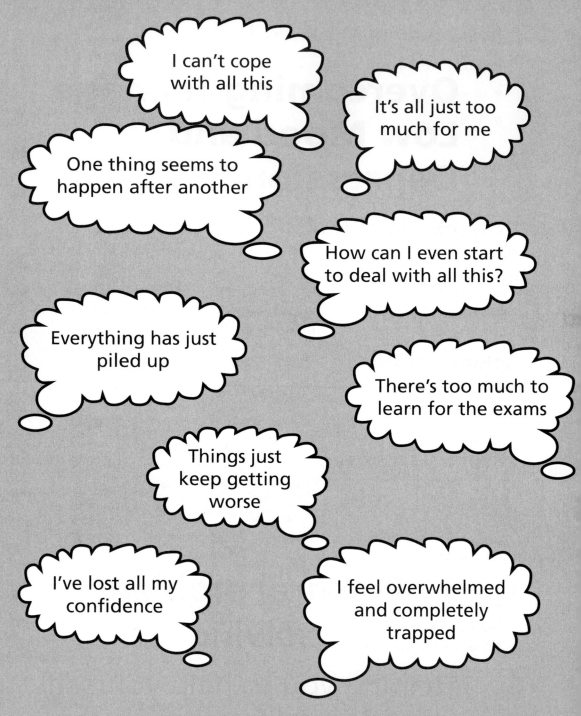

... is this you?

If it is ... this **workbook is for you**.

Overcoming Teenage Low Mood and Depression: A Five Areas Approach

In this workbook you will:

- Learn how practical problems affect our lives

- Identify problems in your own life that you can change

- Read about an example of problem solving in practice and have a chance to apply it to a problem of your own

- Learn how to make slow, steady changes to your life.

How problems affect us

Problems and life difficulties can affect us all. Usually when there's just one problem, we can mostly cope. But when we face a particularly hard problem or a whole lot of smaller things all happen at the same time, we can struggle to cope and we feel overwhelmed.

Before you start

Sometimes problems occur because of things we can't control. But sometimes they're the result of things we could've handled differently. For example, problems in relationships may build up because we've ignored a misunderstanding and kept expecting the other person to do something. But we didn't make it clear what was needed. Or perhaps we didn't respond in ways that would have prevented things worsening at an earlier stage.

 Task

Think about:

1 **Your behaviour**. Do you find that the same kinds of problem occur again and again? If so, is there anything that you keep doing (or not doing) that leads to the problem? If you answered yes, you may find the *Unhelpful things we do* workbook useful.

2 **Other people's behaviour**. Sometimes, other people have to change for our problems to improve. This is particularly so when we're children and teenagers, because we depend on others for our care. Sometimes the person or people who need to change simply can't make the changes that are needed at this time. If you want to think about asking people around you about changing, the *Being assertive* and *Ideas for families and friends* workbooks may help. Also, take a look at the ways of getting further help listed in the *Understanding why I feel as I do* workbook.

It's important to know that many sources of help (for example your general practitioner (GP) or a mental health worker) can keep whatever you tell them confidential (that means not telling your problem to anyone else). The **only exception** to this would be if they hear that you or another young person are seriously at risk of harm from another person. Even then, what will need to be told to whom should be discussed with you first.

How to tackle problems

By approaching your problems one step at a time, it is possible to begin tackling them.

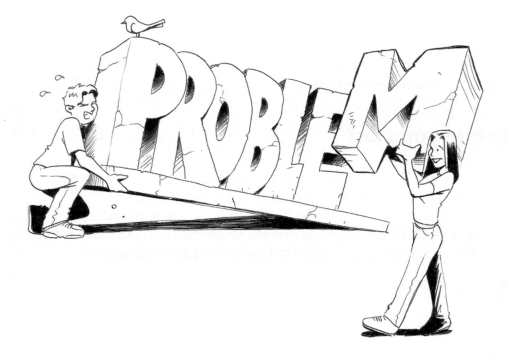

- Approach each problem separately in turn.

- Define the problem clearly.

- Break down seemingly enormous and unmanageable problems into smaller parts that are then easier to solve.

The seven steps to problem solving

Step 1: Identify and define your problem as clearly as possible

Example: Mark's practical problem

Mark's problem is that he isn't confident about being with other people at school any more. Mark needs to break down his problem into some **smaller steps**. These will all then slowly add up to help him sort out his larger problem.

Example: Breaking it down into smaller parts

To identify a better first target Mark needs to answer the question 'Exactly how is this problem going to affect me tomorrow and this week?' By answering this question, he can define more clearly the problem he wants to tackle first as:

I'm scared a group of boys will threaten me when I walk down the corridor to registration tomorrow.

 Is this a small, focused problem I can tackle?

Yes ☑   No ☐

So this is a good first target for Mark to tackle. Sorting out his problem with getting to registration tomorrow won't solve all Mark's confidence problems, but it can be a useful first step. It will be focused enough to be possible, and big enough to move him forwards.

Step 2: Think up as many solutions as possible to achieve your first goal

One problem that often faces us when we feel overwhelmed by practical problems is that we can't see a way out. It can seem hard to even start tackling the problem.

One way around this is to try to step back from the problem and see if any other solutions are possible. This approach is called **brainstorming**. The more solutions that you can think of, the more likely it is that a good one will emerge.

Key point

You can even include ridiculous ideas at first as you are just trying to get yourself to start thinking more flexibly.

The idea of brainstorming is to try come up with **as many ideas as possible.** And from them, you should be able to identify a realistic, practical and achievable solution for overcoming your problem.

Example: Mark's problem – possible solutions
(Including ridiculous ideas at first)

- Ignore the problem completely – it may go away
- Hire a minder
- Offer them money
- Learn a martial art and turn the tables
- Try to be friendly to them
- Speak to my class tutor
- Ask anyone else I see to protect me.

Step 3: Look at the pros and cons of each possible solution

Mark writes down the pros and cons of his solutions.

Suggestion	Pros (advantages)	Cons (disadvantages)
Ignore the problem completely – it may go away	Easier in the short term and I don't have to think about it. They may not even be there tomorrow	The problems will worsen in the long term. It's been going on for ages and they said they'd hit me next time I 'wasn't respectful'
Hire a minder	Might scare them off	There's no one I can think of and I don't have money to pay. It wouldn't help my confidence
Offer them money	This may persuade them to be friendly tomorrow	I'm short of cash and also it might make them think bullying me pays well so they do it more
Learn a martial art and turn the tables	I'd look pretty cool	No way I can do that by tomorrow and anyway they'd still overpower me between them
Try to be friendly to them	They may be friendly	They may not want to be friendly and keep threatening me. I may end up crying again like last time
Speak to my class tutor	I know Mr Cox helped Helen with something like this once	I'd feel embarrassed talking to him, especially as I'm a bloke. He'll think I'm pathetic
Ask anyone else I see to protect me	They might help	It seems quite scary to do this. They might not want to help or might think I'm useless

Step 4: Choose one of the solutions

Mark tries to choose the option that will make a sensible first step in achieving his goal. His chosen solution should be **realistic** and **likely to succeed**. Mark makes his decision after looking at all the answers in Step 3.

Example: Mark's choice

Mark decides to arrange to talk to Mr Cox. His other suggestions might also have worked, but this one seems to be a reasonable solution for him as he knows that Mr Cox helped Helen. If he hadn't been aware of this, then choosing one of the other options would have seemed better.

Now see if you can answer 'Yes' to the first three **questions for effective change** below:

Q Will it be **useful** for changing how I am?

Yes ☑   No ☐

Is it a **specific** task so that I will know when I have done it?

Yes ☑   No ☐

Is it something that is realistic, practical and achievable?

Yes ☑   No ☐

If you answered 'Yes' to all three questions your chosen step should help start you off.

Step 5: Plan the steps needed to carry out your chosen solution

Example: Mark's plan

I could catch Mr Cox at the end of registration and ask if I can talk to him today about something. I shall ask if I can see him after lunch as I generally feel less tense in the afternoons, less easily upset and also more confident then. I will need to explain to him that I have to speak to him today as I should have spoken to him before tomorrow. I will try to write down and practise in advance what I will say to him.

Next, Mark needs to apply the **questions for effective change** to his plan to check how practical and achievable it is.

Q Is the planned solution one that:

- Will be useful for understanding or changing how I am?

  Yes ☑   No ☐

- Is a specific task so that I will know when I have done it?

  Yes ☑   No ☐

- Is realistic, practical and achievable?

  Yes ☑   No ☐

- Makes clear what I am going to do and when I am going to do it?

  Yes ☑   No ☐

- Is an activity that won't be easily blocked or prevented by practical problems?

  Yes ☑   No ☐

- Will help me to learn useful things even if it doesn't work out perfectly?

  Yes ☑   No ☐

Mark needs to answer 'Yes' to all of the questions. If he can't, he will need to think of some changes he could make to improve his plan.

Key point

Part of this planning should include Mark having a planned response of how to react if his request is turned down.

What if it doesn't work out? Mark writes his plan here:

> If it doesn't work out I'll definitely be disappointed. I'll need to find another solution before tomorrow by going back to my list of brainstorming ideas. I'll probably try to talk to another member of staff and ask their advice.

Step 6: Carry out the plan

Example: Mark carries out his first step

Mark waits at the end of registration to see Mr Cox as planned. While he's waiting, he feels quite scared. He thinks that Mr Cox 'will humiliate me – maybe make me explain myself in front of everyone and turn down my request'.

Mark decides to challenge these fears and carries on waiting anyway. Several people seem to want to talk to Mr Cox too. When Mark gets a chance to speak, Mr Cox does not hear at first as someone else tries to talk at the same time. Mark is surprised by this and is quite taken aback. He becomes flustered and immediately stops talking.

Mark's immediate thought is: 'I'm really pathetic – I can't even do this.' But in the next few minutes, he is able to challenge this thought. He remembers that this sort of thing happens a lot at the end of registration. He just needs to be ready for it next time. He decides to learn from what happened and tries again (but more loudly) when next time there's a lull in the conversation. He finds that Mr Cox is polite and friendly. His anxiety begins to drop as he makes his request. Mr Cox agrees immediately without asking Mark to give any reasons for his request.

That afternoon, when Mark goes to see Mr Cox he begins to feel quite scared again. He is almost convinced he will be rejected. Importantly, again Mark plucks up courage and decides to challenge these fears and go and see Mr Cox anyway, in spite of his worries.

This is the best way to experiment and test out how true our fears are – by acting against them and seeing what happens.

When Mark arrives, he's surprised to find Mr Cox is friendly and welcoming. Mr Cox shuts his door carefully so that their discussion is confidential. After Mark has explained the problem, he is surprised that Mr Cox thanks him for being helpful as several other people have also been threatened by the same boys and the school is wanting to monitor the situation carefully. Because of this Mr Cox would like to watch discreetly from a distance tomorrow morning as Mark comes to registration. He will step in immediately if any problems arise. Mark agrees, and is happy with how things went. His fears were not correct. A particular bonus is that he has been offered help that is discreet and so won't embarrass him.

Step 7: Review your learning

Mark's review

Q Was my selected solution successful?

Yes ☑   No ☐

Q Did it help me to tackle my target problem?

Yes ☑   No ☐

Q Did I have any problems using this approach?

Yes ☐   No ☑

What have I learnt from doing this?

> Things went smoothly the second time I spoke up. Even when the problem arose when I shut up on the first occasion, I learned from it and didn't give up. I changed my plan by speaking louder the next time. By sticking with it and not giving up I sorted out my problem, and also realised that my worries were quite wrong.

In this example, Mark's plan went smoothly. Even if there were any problems, he could've learned from them and used them to improve his next attempt to solve the problem.

Mark's example shows us how the seven-step approach might be applied to this situation. But it also works for any other day-to-day problem.

Key point

Please note that Mark chose this option of going to Mr Cox because he knew he had previously helped Helen. Even so, sometimes we can over-estimate how likely something is to succeed. If Mark had been turned down he would've been surprised and upset. But remember that he had already thought of a plan (at Step 5) of what he could do if he was turned down.

So even if Mark had been turned down he would have achieved the following:

- He has a clear idea of his target problem that he is going to work on.

- He has a list of other solutions that he could use to tackle the problem. Some of these may well have worked better.

- He has learned an approach he can try again.

- He can take what he has learned and include it in his own review.

- Finally, he can take pride that he has acted against his fear and will be better able to do this again in the future. He will be less trapped by his fears from now on.

Now it's your turn to practise this approach.

My problem solving

Think about how you can begin to tackle the problems you face in your own life. Remember, the aim isn't to change things across the board. Instead the plan is to tackle **one** problem at a time.

Step 1: Identify and define your problem as clearly as possible

The first step to problem solving is making sure that you have identified one target problem. This step is particularly important if you feel overwhelmed by many different kinds of problems.

Checklist of problems you face

Q Family and home: Do these cause problems in my life?

- I have problems getting on with one or more of my parents or carers

    Often ☐ Sometimes ☐ No ☐

- I have problems getting on with another person or people in my family

    Often ☐ Sometimes ☐ No ☐

- One or both of my parents or carers has been absent, left home or gone away

    Often ☐ Sometimes ☐ No ☐

- I am now living separately from some or all of my family

    Often ☐ Sometimes ☐ No ☐

- My family has housing problems (for example too small or may have to leave)

    Often ☐ Sometimes ☐ No ☐

- My family has unemployment (joblessness) or money worries

    Often ☐ Sometimes ☐ No ☐

- I am or we are having problems with neighbours

    Often ☐ Sometimes ☐ No ☐

Q Friends and other relationships: Do these cause problems in my life?

- I have fallen out with one or more of my friends
  Often ☐   Sometimes ☐   No ☐

- There is no one around whom I can really talk to
  Often ☐   Sometimes ☐   No ☐

- Someone or some people important to me have been absent or gone away
  Often ☐   Sometimes ☐   No ☐

- Someone else close to me has physical or mental health problems
  Often ☐   Sometimes ☐   No ☐

- Someone else close to me has drug or alcohol problems
  Often ☐   Sometimes ☐   No ☐

Q School or college: Does this cause problems in my life?

- I have problems with school or college work, exams or tests
  Often ☐   Sometimes ☐   No ☐

- I have problems with attending school or college
  Often ☐   Sometimes ☐   No ☐

- I have recently changed school or college
  Often ☐   Sometimes ☐   No ☐

- I have problems with other people my age at school or college
  Often ☐   Sometimes ☐   No ☐

- I have problems with staff at my school or college
  Often ☐   Sometimes ☐   No ☐

- I am being bullied or picked on
  Often ☐   Sometimes ☐   No ☐

Q Things that have happened in my life. Are any still happening?

- Someone doing or saying things they shouldn't so that I didn't or don't feel safe
  Often ☐   Sometimes ☐   No ☐

- Something else has happened that has really upset me or someone close to me
  Often ☐   Sometimes ☐   No ☐

Write down any other problems you may have.

Look at your list again and identify **one** target area that you will first focus on. This is particularly important if you have ticked many 'Often' or 'Sometimes' boxes in the checklist. It isn't possible to overcome all these problems at once.

My target area

Write down the one problem area you want to work on here.

Key point

Make sure this is an external problem – that is, a problem involving other people, school, etc. rather than a problem with your own thoughts or emotions.

You may find the thought of making changes daunting or impossible. The important thing is to use a **step-by step** approach in which no step seems too large. This first step needs to be something that gets you moving in the right direction.

Ask yourself if you need to break down this problem area into even more smaller more achievable targets? Look at Mark's example on page **167** if in doubt.

Now ask yourself: Is this a good first target? If it isn't, what smaller steps do you need to tackle first? Choose a smaller part of your problem that you would wish to change at the present time.

Key point

Again, remember that this should be an external problem – not something to do with your own thoughts or emotions.

Write your first target here:

Q **Is my chosen problem clear and focused?**
Yes ☐   No ☐

Q **Is it realistic, practical and achievable?**
Yes ☐   No ☐

If you answer 'No' to either question, write down your target problem again.

Q **Is this a realistic target for change?**

Imagine if throughout your life one of your relations has been difficult with you. It's probably unrealistic that your plan should include them changing to suddenly be really easy to get on with.

Instead you could focus on planning how you react to live with them as they are. If they do change that's great. But you have to be realistic that any change they make might be quite small and will take some time.

Step 2: Think up as many solutions as possible of how you can achieve your first goal

Remember, try to **think broadly**. Here are some useful questions to help you to think up possible solutions:

- What advice would I give a friend who was trying to tackle the same problem? Sometimes we can think of solutions for others more easily than for ourselves.

- What ridiculous solutions can I include as well as more sensible ones?

- What helpful suggestions would others (for example family, friends or colleagues at work) make?

- How could I look at the solutions facing me differently? For example, what would you have said before you felt like this, or what might you say about the situation say in five years' time?

- What approaches have I tried in the past in similar circumstances?

  If you feel stuck, sometimes doing this task with someone you trust can be helpful.

Brainstorming my problem

Write down your ideas of possible solutions (and include some ridiculous ideas at first).

Step 3: Look at the pros and cons of each possible solution

The next step is to think about the pros and cons of each possible solution.

My suggestion	Pros (advantages)	Cons (disadvantages)

Step 4: Choose one of the solutions

Try to choose the solution that will make a sensible first step in tackling your problem. It should be realistic and likely to succeed. You should make your decision after looking at all your answers in Step 3.

The kind of solution you are looking for is therefore something that gets you moving in the right direction. This should be small enough to be possible, but big enough to move you forwards. Look at your responses in Step 3. Write your preferred solution here.

Now see if you can answer 'Yes' to the three questions below about your chosen step:

Q Will it be **useful** for changing how I am?

Yes ☐   No ☐

Q Is it a **specific** task so that I will know when I've done it?

Yes ☐   No ☐

Q Is it something that is realistic, practical and achievable?

Yes ☐   No ☐

If you answered 'Yes' to all three questions your chosen step should help start you off.

Step 5: Plan the steps needed to carry out your solution

You need to have a clear plan that will help you to decide exactly **what** you are going to do and **when** you are going to do it. It is useful to **write down** the steps you've planned. This will help you to plan what you're going to do and to think of the possible problems that might arise. Remember to build into your plan some thought about what you will do if the plan doesn't fully succeed.

My plan
Also write ways of tackling any possible blocks that might get in the way. This is the **key part** of the problem-solving process. Be as clear as possible about your plan.

Next, apply the **questions for effective change** to your plan to check how practical and achievable it is.

Q Is my planned task one that:

- Will be useful for understanding or changing how I am?

  Yes ☐   No ☐

- Is a specific task so that I will know when I have done it?

  Yes ☐   No ☐

- Is realistic, practical and achievable?

  Yes ☐   No ☐

- Makes clear **what** I am going to do and **when** I am going to do it?

  Yes ☐   No ☐

- Is an activity that won't be easily blocked or prevented by practical problems?

  Yes ☐   No ☐

- Will help me to learn useful things even if it doesn't work out perfectly?

  Yes ☐   No ☐

You should have answered 'Yes' to each of the questions. If you've answered 'No' to one of the questions, try to change things so that any problems with your plan can be sorted.

You should include planning what you will do if your first step doesn't fully work out. Write your plan of what you can do next if your first step doesn't work out.

What if it doesn't work out?

Step 6: Carry out your plan

Pay attention to your thoughts about what will happen before, during and after you have completed your plan.

Record and rate on a scale of 0 to 100 your thoughts or worries and your level of anxiety before, during and after you do this. Remember that the best way to challenge fears is to act against them.

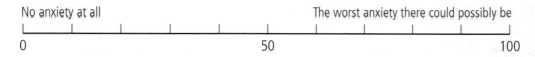

No anxiety at all   The worst anxiety there could possibly be

0   50   100

Now record and rate on a scale of 0 to 100 how much you now believe your previous thoughts or worries. Again remember that the best way to challenge your worries is to act against them

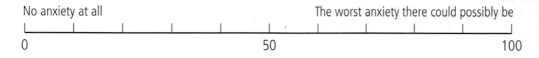

No anxiety at all   The worst anxiety there could possibly be

0   50   100

Step 7: Review your learning

Write down what happened here.

Q Was the approach successful?

Yes ☐ No ☐

Q Did it help improve things?

Yes ☐ No ☐

Q Did I have any problems using this approach?

Yes ☐ No ☐

Q What have I learnt from doing this?

Write down any helpful lessons or information you have learned from what happened. If things didn't go quite as you hoped, try to learn from this.

Q How could you do things differently next time?

If you noticed problems with your plan

Choosing realistic targets for change is important. Were you too ambitious or unrealistic in choosing the target you did? Sometimes a problem-solving approach may be blocked by something unexpected that happens. Perhaps something didn't happen as you planned, or someone reacted in an unexpected way? Try to learn from what happened.

How could you change how you approach the problem to help you make a realistic action plan?

Planning the next steps

Now that you have looked at how your first planned response went, the next step is to plan something else to build on this. You need to think about your **short-term**, **medium-term** and **longer-term** targets. Did your problem-solving plan help you to completely solve the problem? You may need to think of different solutions to tackle the various parts of your problem.

The key is to build one step upon another.

 ### Example: Mark's next steps

Mark's last plan helped him deal with the immediate issue ('I'm scared a group of boys will threaten me when I walk along the corridor to registration tomorrow'). His actions will have helped him tide things over for a time. But there are other things that he also needs to deal with (such as looking at ways of getting back his confidence with people in general).

Use what you have learned to build on what you did. Without a step-by-step approach you may find that although you take some steps forward, they're all in different directions and you lose your focus and motivation.

Many people find this approach takes quite a lot of practice. It may also be tempting to be too ambitious and try to sort everything out all at once.

Key point

Remember large changes can be achieved by moving one step at a time.

Taking slow, sure steps will also boost your confidence. It will increase your sense of being able to deal with the problems you face.

Do

- Continue to plan to change **only** one problem area at a time.
- Break down the problem into smaller parts that each build towards your eventual goal. There can be as many or as few steps as you want in your plan.
- Make a plan to slowly tackle your wider problem in a way that will work for you.
- Be realistic in your goals.
- Write down your plan in detail so that you will be able to put it into practice this week.

Don't

- Choose something that is too big a target to do next.
- Try to start to change too many areas of your life all at once.
- Be negative and think 'nothing can be done'. Try to experiment to find out if this negative thinking is true or helpful.

You can sort out most problems using this approach. Again, remember the main reason why a plan might not work is if you are too ambitious or allow yourself to believe that change is impossible.

Once you have chosen the next step you wish to change, write it down here.

Use the seven-step approach again to work out what to do in detail. You'll find these in a shorter form (as an example and as a worksheet) on pages **190–94** of this workbook.

Summary

In this workbook you have:

- Learnt how practical problems affect our lives
- Learnt how to identify problems in your own life that you can change
- Seen an example of problem solving in practice and had a chance to apply this to one of your own problems
- Learnt how to make slow, steady changes to your life.

Let's look at the whole picture again

After you've been putting this workbook into action in your life for a while, rate the size of your problems again in each of the **five areas**.

Q Overall, do I have (or have I had) problems in Area 1: People and events?

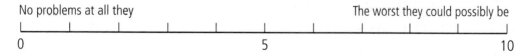

No problems at all they   The worst they could possibly be

0   5   10

Q Overall, do I have problems in Area 2: Altered thinking?

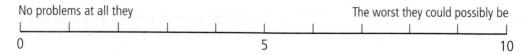

No problems at all they   The worst they could possibly be

0   5   10

Q Overall, do I have problems in Area 3: Altered feelings?

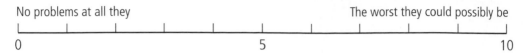

No problems at all they   The worst they could possibly be

0   5   10

Q Overall, do I have problems in Area 4: Altered physical symptoms?

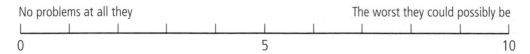

No problems at all they   The worst they could possibly be

0   5   10

Q Overall, do I have problems in Area 5: Altered behaviours?

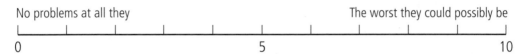

No problems at all they   The worst they could possibly be

0   5   10

Q What have I learnt from this review?

Q What do I want to try next?

Putting into practice what you have learnt

Continue to put into practice what you learn over the next few weeks. Don't try to solve every problem all at once. Plan out what to do at a pace that's right for you. Build changes one step at a time.

Use the blank summary sheet at the end of this workbook to help you plan your changes. If you are stuck or unsure what to do discuss this with someone else.

Don't put off asking for help if you are stuck.

My notes

The seven steps to practical problem solving – worksheet

By working through the seven steps you will learn an approach that will help you to solve your own problems.

Step 1: Identify and define the problem as clearly as possible

Select the problem area you will tackle.

Do you need to break it down into a smaller target that is more practical, realistic and achievable in the next week or so? If yes, write down your new target here.

Step 2: Think up as many solutions as possible of how you can achieve your first goal

Brainstorm: What advice would you give a friend? Include ridiculous ideas as well. What have others said? What would you say in five years' time?

Step 3: Look at the pros and cons of each possible solution

Write down a list of the pluses and minuses of each option.

My suggestion	Pros (advantages)	Cons (disadvantages)

Step 4: Choose one of the solutions

Use your answers in Step 3 to make this choice.

My solution

Step 5: Plan the steps needed to carry out the solution

You'll need to use another sheet of paper for this. Apply the **questions for effective change**.

Q Is the planned activity one that:

1 Will be useful for understanding or changing how I am?

Yes ☐   No ☐

2 Is a specific task so that I will know when I have done it?

Yes ☐   No ☐

3 Is realistic, practical and achievable?

Yes ☐   No ☐

4 Makes clear **what** I am going to do and **when** I am going to do it?

Yes ☐   No ☐

5 Is an activity that won't be easily blocked by practical problems?

Yes ☐   No ☐

6 Will help me to learn useful things even if it doesn't work out perfectly?

Yes ☐   No ☐

Add a plan of what you will do if your solution **doesn't fully work out.**

Step 6: Carry out the plan

Record and rate on a scale of 0 to 100 your thoughts or worries and your level of anxiety before, during and after you do this. Remember that the best way to challenge fears is to act against them.

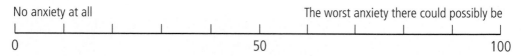

No anxiety at all   The worst anxiety there could possibly be

0   50   100

Now record and rate on a scale of 0 to 100 how much you now believe your previous thoughts or worries. Again remember that the best way to challenge your worries is to act against them

No anxiety at all   The worst anxiety there could possibly be

0   50   100

Step 7: Review your learning

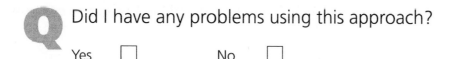 Was my selected approach successful?

Yes ☐   No ☐

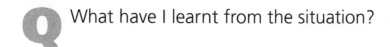 Did I have any problems using this approach?

Yes ☐   No ☐

Q What have I learnt from the situation?

Even if the plan wasn't completely successful, there will be things you would've learnt.

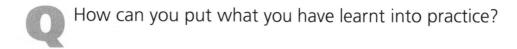 How can you put what you have learnt into practice?

My notes

Overcoming Teenage Low Mood and Depression

A Five Areas Approach

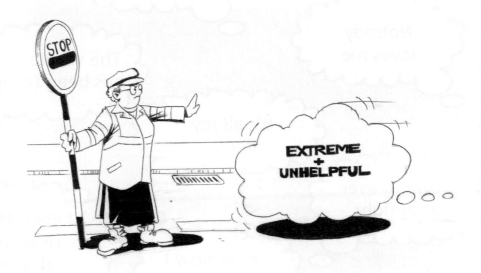

Noticing and changing extreme and unhelpful thinking

Helping you to help yourself

www.livinglifetothefull.com

www.fiveareas.com

Dr Nicky Dummett and Dr Chris Williams

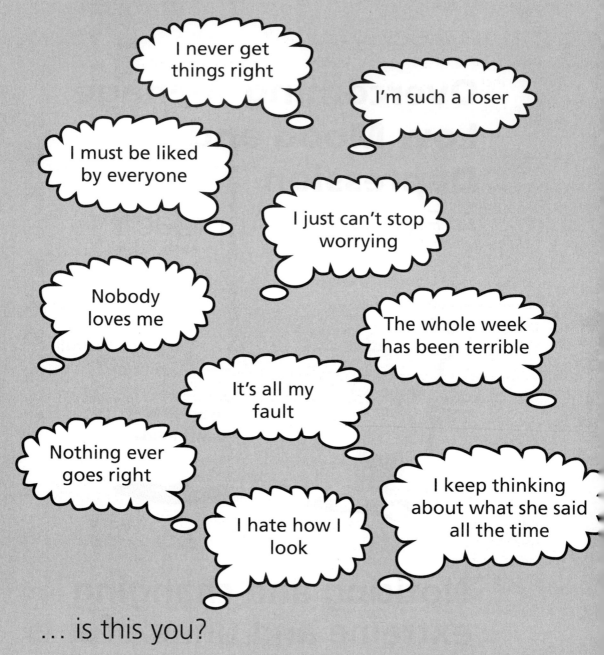

... is this you?

When we feel low or stressed we often start to feel anxious and fearful – this makes us feel tense and stressed. We start to have unhappy negative thoughts – these make us feel **low and sad**. We also start to have frustrated angry thoughts about ourselves, our situation and sometimes others, such as our friends and relatives.

We may have **all sorts of unhelpful thoughts** about how we feel, our current situation and our future.

In this workbook you will:

- Learn how to recognise patterns of extreme and unhelpful thinking that worsen how you feel

- Learn to change this sort of thinking so it's less upsetting.

The first step in changing unhelpful thinking is to start noticing how **common** it is in your life.

Frustration, anger, distress, shame, guilt and feeling down are often linked to the unhelpful patterns of thinking – the unhelpful thinking styles.

Checklist of the unhelpful thinking styles

Unhelpful thinking style	Some typical thoughts	Tick if you have noticed this thinking style recently – even if it's just sometimes
Bias against myself	<ul><li>I'm very self-critical</li><li>I overlook my strengths</li><li>I see myself as not coping</li><li>I don't recognise my achievements</li><li>I knew that would happen to me!</li></ul>	☐
Putting a negative slant on things (negative mental filter)	<ul><li>I see things through dark-tinted glasses</li><li>I see the glass as being half empty rather than half full</li><li>Whatever I've done in the week, it's never enough to give me a sense of achievement</li><li>I tend to focus on the bad side of everyday situations</li></ul>	☐
Having a gloomy view of the future (make negative predictions)	<ul><li>I think that things will stay bad or get even worse</li><li>I tend to think that things will go wrong</li><li>If one thing goes wrong I often think that everything will go wrong</li><li>I'm always looking for the next thing to fail</li></ul>	☐

Unhelpful thinking style	Some typical thoughts	Tick if you have noticed this thinking style recently – even if it's just sometimes
Jumping to the very worst conclusion (catastrophising)	• I tend to think that the very worst outcome will happen • I often think that I will fail badly	☐
Having a negative view about how others see me (mind-reading)	• I mind-read what others think of me • I often think that others don't like me or think badly of me without evidence for it	☐
Unfairly taking responsibility for things	• I think I should take the blame if things go wrong • I feel guilty about things that aren't really my fault • I think I'm responsible for everyone else	☐
Making extreme statements or rules	• I use the words 'always' and 'never' a lot to summarise things • If one bad thing happens to me I often say 'just typical' because it seems this always happens • I make myself a lot of 'must', 'should' 'ought' or 'got to' rules	☐

Almost everyone has these sorts of thoughts each and every day. They're often present and can affect how we feel.

This doesn't mean that:

• You think like this **all** the time.

• You have to notice **all** of the unhelpful thinking styles.

How do these patterns of thinking affect us?

Often we believe in these kinds of thoughts just because they 'feel' true. And this is because of how we're feeling in ourselves. We may forget to check out how true these thoughts really are.

Usually when we notice these kinds of thoughts we may feel a little upset but then quickly move on and carry on with life. But there are times when we're more prone to these thoughts and find them harder to dismiss. For example, when we have some problem we're finding hard to cope with or if we're distressed we typically notice these thoughts more often. We may also dwell on them more than usual and find it harder to dismiss them and move on.

What we think can have a powerful effect on us. It affects how we **feel** and what we **do**. So our unhelpful thinking styles lead to:

1 **Mood changes**. We may become more down, guilty, upset, anxious, ashamed, stressed or angry.

2 **Behaviour changes**. Our unhelpful thinking styles strongly affect what we do, so of course we stop doing things. They cause us to avoid doing things that seem scary, or push us into reacting in ways that backfire, such as pushing others away or even drinking too much or using street drugs to cope.

The result is that these **unhelpful thinking styles worsen how you feel**.

 Task

Look at the links between our thoughts, feelings and behaviour in the following examples. In the very last column on the right of the table there is a suggestion that stopping, thinking and reflecting (**before** getting carried away by the thought and just ending up feeling worse*)* could help you see things differently.

> *The different unhelpful thinking styles are common patterns of thinking that can worsen how you feel and affect what you do. They are more common than you may expect at times of distress. Thinking in these extreme ways means that you're only looking at part of the picture. Because of this, these thinking styles are **often not true**.*

Example: Dealing with unhelpful thinking

Situation	Unhelpful thinking style	Altered feelings	Altered behaviour
You are walking down the road and someone you know walks past and says nothing. They don't smile or meet your eye – just walk by **Thought:** *There's poor Paul – he looks really distracted and upset. I hope he's okay*	This is normal concern for others. No unhelpful thinking style	Concern for Paul	You turn round and catch up with Paul to say hello. Paul looks a little surprised to begin with and says he didn't see you. You get chatting and have a helpful talk. At the end you both agree to meet for lunch after the shopping to catch up **Stop, think and reflect:** *I'm really pleased I spoke to him. He is feeling upset. It was nice to talk – and he seemed pleased too. He suggested we meet up for lunch which is good because it says to me that he wants to see me*
You are walking down the road and someone you know walks past and says nothing. They don't smile or meet your eye – just walk by. **Thought:** *They don't like me*	Unhelpful thinking styles: • Mind-reading: they don't like you • Jump to the worst conclusion • Bias against yourself	Low/down and upset Anxious in case you meet again	• Feel so down you just go home • Avoid them in future **Stop, think and reflect:** *You never checked out that this was the real reason. Maybe they just didn't see you?*
You are at a supermarket checkout and hear someone behind you tut as you pack the bags **Thought:** *I'm being too slow. They're annoyed with me*	Unhelpful thinking styles: • Bias against yourself (blame yourself) • Mind-reading	• Anxiety • Perhaps anger – how dare they!	• If anxious: maybe speed up packing – fumble and start to drop things. Make all sorts of apologies • If angry: perhaps slow down the packing, stare at them or pass a sarcastic comment **Stop, think and reflect:** *Maybe they were tutting at something else. Maybe they'd forgotten to pick up the apples. Maybe their teeth don't fit!*

Noticing extreme and unhelpful thinking

The next step is to practise ways of **noticing** extreme and unhelpful thinking. This is the first and most important step in beginning to change how you think. Once you can notice these patterns to your thinking you can step back and choose not to have such thinking patterns.

The examples on the following pages will help you begin to see how extreme thinking may affect how you feel and what you do.

Mark's Five Areas thought review of a time when he felt worse

Life situation, relationships and practical problems
- What time of day is it?
- Where am I?
- Who am I with?
- What am I doing?
- What has been said or happened?

Lunchtime. In dining hall by myself. Saw three of my friends chatting on the other side of hall and wanted to go to speak to them

Altered thinking
- What went through my mind at the time?
- Any thoughts about:
  Me or how I am coping?
  The worst that could happen?
  How others see me?
  My own body, behaviour or performance?
  Any memories or mental pictures?

I won't have anything to say
They won't be interested in speaking to me

Altered feelings
- How do I feel emotionally at the time?
- Am I anxious, ashamed, depressed, angry or guilty?

Anxious

Altered physical symptoms
Note down any strong physical reactions I notice at the time

Feel tense, heart speeded up, breathing a little faster, and a little sweaty

Altered behaviour
- What did I do differently?
- Did I stop doing what I was doing, or start doing something different?

Turned around and left the dining room and went and sat alone outside

Example: Mark's unhelpful thinking

Mark is feeling lonely. He sees his friends chatting together on the other side of the room. He wants to go to speak to them but starts to feel anxious about how it will go. He worries he won't have anything to say and that his friends wouldn't be interested in speaking to him. He feels physically tense too – he has a rapid heart and breathing (common in anxiety) and feels sweaty. He turns around and leaves the room. This prevents him knowing that he would've been very welcome and would've had a good chat with his mates leading on to a game of football that he would have enjoyed. Because of his fears he never did that and instead sat alone 'feeling like a fool' afterwards for not having gone over.

Completing your own thought review

Now let's look in detail at a particular time when you felt worse.

First, try to really think yourself back into a situation in the past few days when your mood unhelpfully changed. To begin with **don't choose a time when you have felt very distressed.** Instead, pick an occasion when you noticed **some** moderate upset, tension, symptoms, anger or guilt. Try to be as slow as you can when you think back through the situation so that you're as accurate as you can be. Stop, think and reflect as you go through the five different areas that can be affected.

Before you start – what to do if you find it's hard to even think about the upsetting situation

Sometimes it can feel distressing going back over a time when we have felt worse. That's why it's important to begin by choosing a time that wasn't so distressing that just looking at it in depth will make you feel too upset.

The whole idea here is to make you feel able to change such thoughts and to feel less distressed. Sometimes our concerns, worries and fears can feel terrifying and too much to look at all in one go. So if you feel this way, the key is to slowly start practising this approach with less upsetting thoughts to begin with.

Start to notice the thoughts that link in with feeling **somewhat or moderately upset**. Work with these moderately upsetting thoughts first, and use the rest of the workbook to practise changing these. You can slowly work up to more upsetting thoughts later when you are feeling more confident.

🖈 Task

Use the blank five areas diagram on page **205** to go through what you noticed in each of the five areas.

Think about:

1 Events and people

- Where were you?

- What time of day was it?

- Who else was there?

- What was said?

- What happened?

Write the answers in Box 1 of the blank five areas diagram on page **205**.

2 Altered thinking

- What went through your mind at the time?

- How did you see yourself?

- How you were coping? For example did you have any bias against yourself?

- What did you think was the worst thing that could happen? Were you expecting the worst – that is, catastrophic thinking?

- How did you think others saw you? Were you mind-reading?

- What did you think about your own body, behaviour or performance?

- Were there any painful memories from the past?

- Did you think up any images or pictures in your mind (images can have a powerful effect on how you feel)?

Write down any thoughts you notice in Box 2. **Underline** the most upsetting thought.

3 Altered feelings

- How did you feel emotionally at the time?

- Were you anxious, ashamed, depressed, angry or guilty?

Write these things in Box 3.

4 Altered physical symptoms

You may have had many different physical reactions:

- Feelings of muscle tension, jitteriness or pain in anxiety or anger

- Other anxiety-related symptoms, for example a rapid heart and breathing, feeling hot, sweaty and clammy

- Poor concentration and feelings of low energy, pressure or even pain.

Write these things in Box 4.

5 Altered behaviour

Remember that this can be any of the following:

- Reduced activity: where you reduce or stop doing what you had planned to do

- Avoidance or escape: where you suddenly feel anxious and avoid doing something or going somewhere or escape from a situation without staying to see if the thing you fear really happens

- Unhelpful behaviours: where you try to block how you feel by acting in ways that may make you feel better in the short term but backfire in the longer term.

Write these things in Box 5.

At the same time, you may also have noticed other more helpful responses

My Five Areas thought review of a time when I felt worse

📌 **Task**

Please write in your experience in all five areas.

Box 1: People and events
- What time of day is it?
- Where am I?
- Who am I with?
- What am I doing?
- What has been said or happened?

Box 2: Altered thinking
- What went through my mind at the time?
- Any thoughts about:
  - How I am coping?
  - The worst that could happen?
  - How others see me?
  - My own body, behaviour or performance?
  - Any memories or mental pictures?

Underline the thought that is the most upsetting

Box 3: Altered feelings
- How do I feel emotionally at the time?
- Am I anxious, ashamed, depressed, angry or guilty?

Box 4: Altered physical symptoms
Note down any strong physical reactions I notice at the time

Box 5: Altered behaviour
- What did I do differently?
- Did I stop doing what I was doing, or start doing something different?

Overcoming Teenage Low Mood and Depression: A Five Areas Approach   © Dr Nicky Dummet and Dr Chris Williams (2008)

The Five Areas model shows that **what a person thinks** about a situation or problem may **affect how they feel** physically and emotionally, and also may lead them to alter **what they do** (altered behaviour).

What you think ———▶ affects how you feel

What you think ———▶ affects what you do

Q **Does your thought review show this?**
Yes ☐ No ☐

You will find a blank Five Areas assessment sheet at the end of this workbook. Copy this so you can practise this approach.

At first, many people find it can be quite hard to notice their unhelpful thinking. Doing this kind of thought review can help you to begin to practise how to notice your thinking. Over time you'll find that this becomes easier to do. The best way of becoming aware of your extreme and unhelpful thinking is to try to notice times when your mood unhelpfully alters (for example at times when you feel upset), and then to ask 'What is going through my mind right now?'

Remember, we all have all kinds of thoughts during the day. The thoughts we need to especially focus on changing are those that are:

- **Extreme**: that is, they show one of the unhelpful thinking styles

and are also

- **Unhelpful**: that is, they worsen how we feel and/or unhelpfully affect what we do.

Changing our extreme and unhelpful thoughts

The following steps are a **proved way of changing thoughts** that are extreme and unhelpful. You can use as many or as few of the following steps as you need. Just stop when you feel you can move on from the thought.

Tackling the extreme and unhelpful thoughts

1 Label the thought as 'just one of those unhelpful thoughts', rather than 'the truth'

2 Stop think and reflect – don't get caught up in it.

3 Move on – act against it. Don't be put off from what you were going to do.

4 Respond by giving yourself a truly caring response.

Try to act like a scientist:

5 Put the thought under a microscope and ask yourself the seven thought challenge questions.

These steps are described below. Before you start, record how much you believe the extreme and unhelpful thought now:

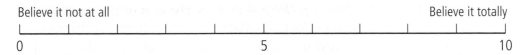

Believe it not at all   Believe it totally

0   5   10

Step 1: Label it as 'just one of those unhelpful thoughts'

When you feel upset, use the list below to tick the unhelpful thinking patterns that are present at that time.

Unhelpful thinking style	Tick if your thought(s) showed this pattern at that time
Am I being my own worst critic? (Biased against yourself)	☐
Am I focusing on the bad in situations? (A negative mental filter)	☐
Am I making negative predictions about the future? (A gloomy view of the future)	☐
Am I jumping to the very worst conclusion? (Catastrophising)	☐
Am I second-guessing that others see me badly without checking if it's actually true? (Mind-reading)	☐
Am I taking unfair responsibility for things that aren't really my fault or taking all the blame?	☐
Am I using unhelpful 'must' or 'should' or 'ought' or 'got to' statements? (Making extreme statements or setting impossible standards)	☐

If the thought doesn't show one of the unhelpful thinking styles then you should stop here.

Step 2: Stop, think and reflect: don't get caught up in it

Simply **noticing** that you're having an unhelpful thinking style can be a powerful way of getting rid of it.

- Label the upsetting thought as **just another** of those unhelpful or even silly thoughts. These are just a part of what happens when we're upset. It will go away and lose its power. It's part of distress – it's not the true picture. You could say to the thought 'I've found you out – I'm not going to play that game again!' or 'Thanks for your input. I'll get back to you at a later stage'.

- Allow the thought to **just be**. Don't allow yourself to get caught up in it. Don't bother trying to challenge the thought, or argue yourself out of it. Like a celebrity, such thoughts love attention. They're just not worth your attention. Allow them to **just be**. Take a mental step back from the thought as if observing it from a distance. Move your mind on to other more helpful things such as the future or recent things you have done well, or even better on to the task in hand.

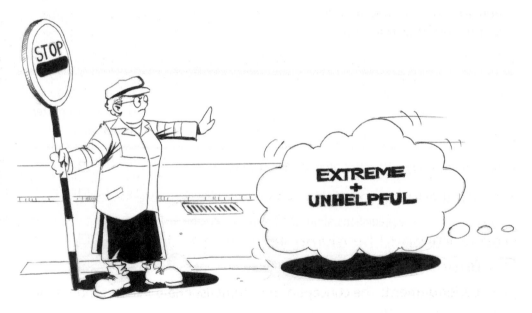

Step 3: Move on. Act against it: don't be put off from what you were going to do

Unhelpful thinking worsens how you feel and unhelpfully alters what you do. The thought may push you to:

- Stop, reduce or avoid doing something you were going to do. This leads to a loss of pleasure and achievement. In the longer term it will restrict your life and undermine your confidence.

- Cause you to feel you must do something, such as drinking, that is actually unhelpful. It ends up backfiring and worsening how you or others feel.

Make an **active choice** not to allow this to happen again. This often means acting against the thought. Choose to react helpfully rather than unhelpfully. Choose not to be bullied into changing what you do by the thought.

To stand up to the bully try these three dos and don'ts.

Do

- **Keep doing** what you planned to do anyway. Keep to your plan. Stay active.

- **Face your fears**. Act against thoughts that tell you that things are too scary and you should avoid things. By creating a step-by-step approach you can overcome these fears. See the *Restarting things we've avoided* workbook.

- **Experiment**. If a thought says don't do something – do it. If a thought says you won't enjoy going to that party, try going to see whether or not you do.

Don't

- Get pushed into not doing things by the thoughts.

- Let fear rule your life.

- Block how you feel with drink or even drugs or by seeking reassurance.

Step 4: Respond by giving yourself a truly caring response

(**Acknowledgement:** The concept of the 'compassionate mind' response was developed by Professor Paul Gilbert.)

If a friend was troubled by a thought or worry, you would offer words of advice to soothe and encourage them. Imagine you have the best friend in the world. Someone who is totally on your side, totally loving and totally caring. What words of advice and encouragement would they say to you? Write their caring advice here.

Q What would someone who wholly and totally loved me say?

Think about this – choose to apply their words in your own situation. Trust what they say. Allow that trust to wash over you and take away the troubling thoughts.

You might choose a close friend or relative, or perhaps a famous person from literature, or, if you have a religious faith, someone from your scriptures. Whoever you choose you need to be aware that the response will be unconditionally positive, caring and supportive.

Example: Mark's caring thoughts

Mark chooses his gran. He thinks back to what she would have said. These are words of support and love: 'You know we all love you Mark. People often lose their confidence when they feel upset. Don't you worry that you didn't approach your friends this time – it's not worth upsetting yourself about. You can always have a chat with them later. They'll be pleased to see you – just you see.'

Step 5: Ask the thought these seven thought challenge questions

Our upsetting thoughts are often incorrect and untrue. Pretend you're a scientist, and look at the thought in a logical way.

The questions you need to ask are:

1 What would I tell a friend who said the same thing?

2 Am I basing this on how I feel rather than on the facts?

3 What would other people say?

4 Am I looking at the whole picture?

5 Does it really matter so much?

6 What would I say about this looking back six months in the future?

7 Do I apply one set of standards to myself and another to others?

Each of these questions helps you take a step back and look at the thought or situation differently.

Taking what works for you

When you use the approach described in this workbook, you'll find that different parts may well work better for you. Use those questions and responses and build them in to your own reaction when you notice upsetting thoughts. Remember, practising will really help.

Also **discussing** your thoughts, fears and concerns with others can sometimes help you get them into a **different perspective.**

Finally, make an overall summary of all the information you have about the upsetting thought.

How much do I believe it now?

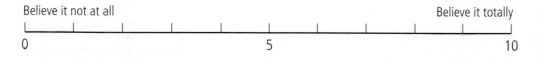

Believe it not at all   Believe it totally

0   5   10

Summary

In this workbook you have:

- Learnt how to notice patterns of extreme and unhelpful thinking that worsen how you feel

- Learnt how to change this kind of thinking so it's less upsetting.

The approach you have worked through will work for any unhelpful thoughts that make you feel worse. By labelling, stepping back from and challenging these thoughts, you will begin to change the way you see yourself, the way things are right now and in the future.

Let's look at the whole picture again

After you have been putting this workbook into action in your life for a while, rate the size of your problems again in each of the **five areas**.

Q Overall, do I have (or have I had) problems in Area 1: People and events?

No problems at all   The worst they could possibly be

0   5   10

Q Overall, do I have problems in Area 2: Altered thinking?

No problems at all   The worst they could possibly be

0   5   10

Q Overall, do I have problems in Area 3: Altered feelings?

No problems at all   The worst they could possibly be

0   5   10

Q Overall, do I have problems in Area 4: Altered physical symptoms?

No problems at all   The worst they could possibly be

0   5   10

Q Overall, do I have problems in Area 5: Altered behaviours?

No problems at all   The worst they could possibly be

0   5   10

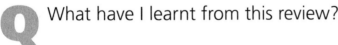 What have I learnt from this review?

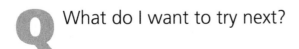 What do I want to try next?

Putting into practice what you have learnt

You will find blank thought practice worksheets at the end of this workbook. Please copy them if you need more. You can also download more sheets from the **www.fiveareas.com** website.

Getting the most from the thought worksheets

To get the most from the worksheets:

● Practise using the approach whenever you notice your mood is changing unhelpfully. With practice you'll find it easier to notice and change your extreme and unhelpful thinking.

● Try to notice and challenge your unhelpful thoughts **as soon as possible** after you notice your mood change.

● If you can't do this immediately, try to think yourself back into the situation so that you are as clear as possible in your answers later on when you do this task.

● With practice you'll find that you can take the most effective parts of the worksheets for you and use them to help you in everyday life.

My notes

Practice sheets

My thought review of a time when I felt worse

Please write in your thoughts in all five areas.

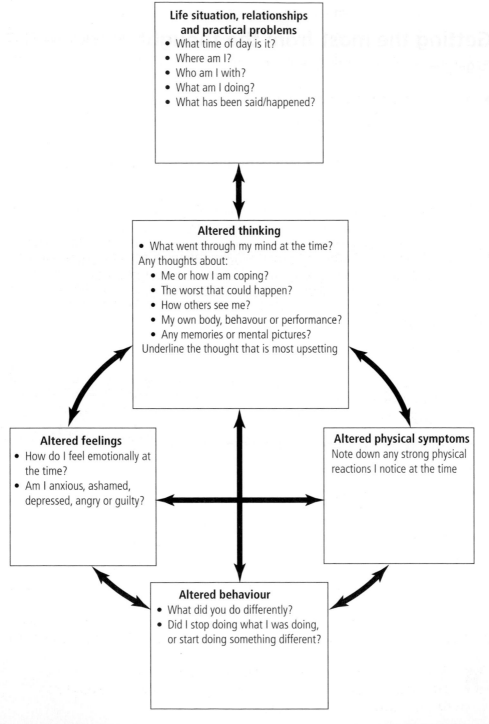

Life situation, relationships and practical problems
- What time of day is it?
- Where am I?
- Who am I with?
- What am I doing?
- What has been said/happened?

Altered thinking
- What went through my mind at the time?
Any thoughts about:
  - Me or how I am coping?
  - The worst that could happen?
  - How others see me?
  - My own body, behavour or performance?
  - Any memories or mental pictures?
Underline the thought that is most upsetting

Altered feelings
- How do I feel emotionally at the time?
- Am I anxious, ashamed, depressed, angry or guilty?

Altered physical symptoms
Note down any strong physical reactions I notice at the time

Altered behaviour
- What did you do differently?
- Did I stop doing what I was doing, or start doing something different?

Summary: The key steps of the thought review

Thought review overview: Try to use the responses below that work for you.

Label the thought as 'just one of those unhelpful thoughts'.

- Am I being my own worst critic? (Bias against yourself)
- Am I focusing on the bad in situations? (A negative mental filter)
- Am I making negative predictions about the future? (A gloomy view of the future)
- Am I jumping to the very worst conclusion? (Catastrophising)
- Am I second-guessing that others see me badly without actually checking if it's actually true? (Mind-reading)
- Am I taking unfair responsibility for things that aren't really my fault/taking all the blame?
- Am I using unhelpful 'must', 'should', 'ought' and 'got to' statements? (Making extreme statements or setting impossible standards)

Stop, think and reflect: Don't get caught up in the thought.

Move on: don't be put off from what you were going to do. Keep active. Face your fears. Keep to your plan. Respond helpfully. Don't be bullied. Act against the upsetting thought and see what happens.

Give yourself a **truly caring response** – for example what would someone who loved you wholly and totally say?

Ask the thought these seven thought challenge questions:

- What would I tell a friend who said the same thing?
- Am I basing this on how I feel rather than the facts?
- What would other people say?
- Am I looking at the whole picture?
- Does it really matter so much?
- What would I say about this looking back six months in the future?
- Do I apply one set of standards to myself and another to others?

Finally, make a summary of everything you have learned. **Remember:** This process takes time and practise to build your confidence in using the approach.

 A downloadable credit-card-sized version of this summary is available free of charge from the Living Life to the Full website (**www.livinglifetothefull.com**).

Overcoming Teenage Low Mood and Depression

A Five Areas Approach

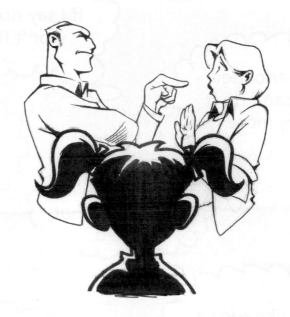

Being assertive

Helping you to help yourself
www.livinglifetothefull.com
www.fiveareas.com

Dr Nicky Dummett and Dr Chris Williams

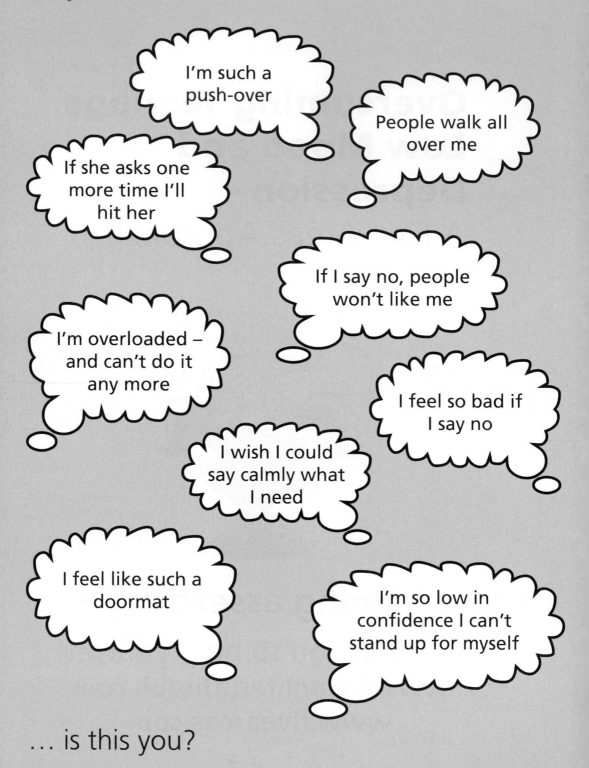

… is this you?

If it is … this **workbook is for you**.

> # In this workbook you will:
>
> - Learn about the differences between passive behaviour, aggressive behaviour and assertive behaviour
> - Learn the rules of assertiveness and how you can put them into practice in everyday situations.

What is assertiveness?

Assertiveness is being able to:

- Stand up for yourself
- Making sure your opinions and feelings are considered
- Not letting other people always get their way.

Key point

You can be assertive **without being forceful or rude**.

So assertiveness means stating clearly what you expect and making sure that what you want is considered **as well as** what other people want.

You can **learn and practise to be** assertive. By practising being assertive, you'll become more aware of your own needs.

Dealing with difficult situations

At some time in our life, all of us, however confident we are, find it hard to deal with certain situations. For example:

- Dealing with unhelpful shop assistants
- Asking someone to return something they have borrowed
- Reacting to angry people in the classroom
- Letting our family or friends know how we feel and what we need
- Saying no to other people's demands.

Often we deal with these situations by losing our temper, by saying nothing or by **giving in**. This may leave us feeling unhappy, angry or out of control. But we still may not actually solve the problem. Sometimes we **dig our heels in** and become very irritable towards everyone else.

How can you become more assertive?

As we grow we learn to relate to others from our parents, teachers and friends. We also get influenced by other things such as television and magazines. Sometimes our confidence is worn away, for example by being bullied or ridiculed at school or criticised within the family. And so we may learn **to react passively or aggressively**.

The good news is that although we may have learned to react passively or aggressively in life, we can learn to become more assertive by using **assertiveness skills**.

Let's first look at what happens when we behave aggressively or passively.

Key elements of passive behaviour

Behaving passively means:

- Always saying 'Yes'
- Not letting others know about our feelings, needs, rights and opinions
- Always choosing others' needs over our own.

Usually people behave passively to **avoid conflict** at all times and to **please others**. This kind of behaviour is driven by a fear of not wanting to upset others or have others not like us. But in the longer term this makes us feel worse.

Our passive behaviour also causes others to become irritated and have a lack of respect for us. They may take us for granted and increasingly expect us to drop everything to help them.

Key elements of aggressive behaviour

Aggression is the opposite of assertiveness.

We are being aggressive when:

- We don't have respect for other people

- We demand things in an angry or threatening way

- We think our own needs are more important than those of others. We ignore other people's needs and think they have little or nothing to contribute.

The aim of aggression is to win, even at the expense of others.

 Task

Q Try to think of a time when someone else has been aggressive towards you and ignored your opinions. How did it make you feel about them and yourself? Write down your feelings here.

Overall, in the longer term being aggressive causes problems for us and for the people around us.

Whether we have problems of aggression or being passive there is a cure. It's called 'assertive communication'.

Key elements of assertive communication

Assertiveness means:

- We let others know about our feelings, needs, rights and opinions while maintaining respect for other people

- We can express our feelings in a direct, honest and appropriate way

- We realise it's possible for us to stand up for our rights in such a way that we don't disregard another person's rights at the same time.

Assertiveness is **not about winning** but about being able to walk away feeling that we put across what we wanted to say.

Task

Q Try to think about a time when someone else has been assertive with you and respected your opinion. How did you feel about them and yourself?

About me – I felt:

About them – I felt:

Benefits of assertive communication

Assertiveness is an **attitude** towards yourself and others that is helpful and honest. When we're being assertive, we ask for what we want:

- Directly and openly
- Appropriately, respecting our opinions and rights and expecting others to do the same
- Confidently without undue anxiety.

We try not to:

- Disregard other people's rights
- Expect other people to magically know what we want
- Freeze with anxiety and avoid problems.

Being assertive improves our self-confidence and others' respect for us.

The rules of assertiveness

The following 12 rules can help you live your life more assertively.

I have the right to:

- Respect myself – who I am and what I do

- Recognise my own needs as an individual – that is, separate from what's expected of me in particular roles, such as 'brother', 'sister', 'partner', 'son', 'daughter'

- Make clear 'I' statements about how I feel and what I think; for example, 'I feel very uncomfortable with your decision'

- Allow myself to make mistakes, recognising that it's normal to make mistakes

- Change my mind, if I choose

- Ask for 'think it over' time. For example, when people ask you to do something, you have the right to say 'I would like to think it over and I will let you know by the end of the week'

- Allow myself to enjoy my successes – that is, being pleased with what I've done and sharing it with others

- Ask for what I want, rather than hoping someone will notice what I want

- Recognise that I am not responsible for the behaviour of adults

- Respect other people and their right to be assertive and expect the same in return

- Say I don't understand

- Deal with others without depending them for approval.

At the moment, how much do you believe in each of these rules, and do you put them into practice?

I have the right to:	Do I believe this rule is true?		Have I applied this in the last week?	
1 Respect myself	Yes ☐	No ☐	Yes ☐	No ☐
2 Recognise my own needs as an individual independent of others	Yes ☐	No ☐	Yes ☐	No ☐
3 Make clear 'I' statements about how I feel and what I think, for example 'I feel very uncomfortable with your decision'	Yes ☐	No ☐	Yes ☐	No ☐
4 Allow myself to make mistakes	Yes ☐	No ☐	Yes ☐	No ☐
5 Change my mind	Yes ☐	No ☐	Yes ☐	No ☐
6 Ask for 'think it over' time	Yes ☐	No ☐	Yes ☐	No ☐
7 Allow myself to enjoy my successes	Yes ☐	No ☐	Yes ☐	No ☐
8 Ask for what I want, rather than hoping someone will notice what I want	Yes ☐	No ☐	Yes ☐	No ☐
9 Recognise that I am not responsible for the behaviour of adults	Yes ☐	No ☐	Yes ☐	No ☐
10 Respect other people and their right to be assertive and expect the same in return	Yes ☐	No ☐	Yes ☐	No ☐
11 Say I don't understand	Yes ☐	No ☐	Yes ☐	No ☐
12 Deal with others without being dependent on them for approval	Yes ☐	No ☐	Yes ☐	No ☐

You can put these rights into practice to develop assertiveness skills by using many assertiveness techniques. Some of these are described below.

The **first thing** to do is start a conversation.

Starting and maintaining conversations

Sometimes we can feel isolated with no-one around to talk to. We may feel lonely but we lack contact with anyone. There are all sorts of practical things you can do to begin to meet people. For example:

- Making friends through people you know already

- Doing a course or joining a club, for example at your local community hall or a youth club

- Visiting other local places where you can meet others, for example community organisations or your local place of worship. Some local businesses such as post offices, pharmacies and hairdressers also provide a place to talk

- Getting in touch with people you knew but haven't seen for a while. Use e-mail, write a letter or telephone. Arrange to meet if you can.

 Task

Think about some good conversation starters:

- How are you?

- Nice day, isn't it?

- Hi, I'm new here and a little bit nervous.

Key point

Remember – it doesn't matter if you talk about superficial things like the weather or football to begin with.

But if you don't like to do this, think of some **conversation starters in advance**. Good opening questions often begin with the words:

- **What** – What was the meeting like last week? What did you do yesterday?

- **How** – How did you find the concert? How are you? How was the talk?

- **When** – When are you away next? When will we be covering this on the course?

- **Who** – Who came yesterday? Who's that over there?

- **Why** – Why does that happen (or not happen)? Why do we do things this way? Why did that (a political or world event) happen?

Follow up with these **back-up questions**. For example:

- Who came yesterday – did they enjoy it?
- What did they say?
- Did it go well?
- Do you think they'll come back?

Assertiveness techniques you could use

Once you get into conversation, the following assertive techniques will help you to build assertive communication into what you say.

'Broken record'

This works in virtually any situation. First, practise what you want to say by repeating over and over again what you want or need. During the conversation, keep returning to your prepared lines, stating clearly what it is you need or want. Do not be put off by clever arguments or by what the other person says. Once you have prepared the lines you want to say, you can relax. Nothing can defeat this tactic!

Example: Being firm about what you want

Anne: Can I borrow £10 from you?

Paul: I can't lend you any money. I've run out.

Anne: I'll pay you back as soon as I can. I need it desperately. You are my friend aren't you?

Paul: I can't lend you any money.

Anne: I would do the same for you. You won't miss £10.

Paul: I am your friend but I can't lend you any money. I'm afraid I've run out.

Remember:

- Work out beforehand what you want to say.
- Repeat your reply over and over again and stick to what you have decided to say.

Saying 'no'

Many people find that 'no' seems to be one of the hardest words to say. We can find ourselves in situations that we don't want to be in just because we've avoided saying this one simple word.

The images we associate with saying 'no' may prevent us from using the word when we need it. We may be scared of being seen as mean and selfish, or of being rejected by others.

Key point

Saying 'no' can be both important and helpful.

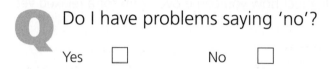

Do I have problems saying 'no'?

Yes ☐   No ☐

If you ticked yes: Try to practise saying 'no' by using the following techniques.

- Be straightforward and honest so that you can make your point effectively. This isn't the same as being rude.

- Tell the person if you are finding it hard.

- Don't apologise and give all sorts of reasons for saying 'no'. It is okay to say 'no' if you don't want to do things.

- Remember that it is better in the long run to be truthful than to breed resentment and bitterness within yourself.

Body language and assertiveness

How we communicate involves more than just words. Our voice tone, how quickly and loudly we speak, eye contact and body posture all contribute to how we come over. When you're being assertive be aware of the non-verbal communications you make as well as the words you say.

Eye contact

- Meet the other person's eyes from time to time.

- Make eye contact – but don't end up staring at the person.

- Try not to look down for long – this may seem a sign of weakness to others.

If you find this hard to do, practise looking just past the person. For example, look at a thing such as a picture on the wall behind them.

You voice

- Try to vary your tone so you come over well.

- Don't be afraid of silence – especially if you've asked a question. You should be aware in advance of the strange change that happens in the physics of time when we feel anxious. If we ask a question we may be tempted to fill any uncomfortable gaps ourselves. Even two seconds can feel too long. Knowing this can be useful so you're prepared to allow a little silence. Likewise you don't need to reply instantly to any question. You're allowed some time to think.

- Think about how quickly or loudly you talk. If you're anxious or angry you may either speed up and gabble words, or slow down so you come over as hesitant. Either extreme will affect how you come over. Aim for a relaxed yet serious manner if you can.

Posture
Think about how you hold your body:

- Try to look up and don't hunch over – which can occur when we feel vulnerable or anxious.

- Keep an appropriate distance ('personal space') between you and the person.

- Don't get too close or this might be seen as aggressive or inappropriate (unless you know the person very well).

Be friendly
Smiling once in a while is okay.

Be relaxed in your body

- Think about how you hold your body. If you're tense or anxious you may clench your fists and frown, which may come over as being aggressive.

- Relax your body. Quickly screen how you're holding your arms and shoulders and try to relax tense muscles.

A word of caution

Don't think you have to suddenly get all of this right straight away. You should make these changes slowly – over many weeks or even months.

You shouldn't get confused because you are concerned about whether you are avoiding eye contact enough. All you need to do is be aware of this and try to occasionally make some small changes in what you do. Experiment and see what works for you.

Trying out being more assertive

Think about the following when you plan to respond assertively. Choose:

- **The right person**. We all know that some people can take even assertive feedback badly. If you know that what you say is likely to be taken badly or that the person will over-react then you need to get some extra help, such as from a close friend or a family member.

- **The right time**. For example, try not to start talking about important things as soon as your mum or dad gets in from work or an evening out. Choose a more relaxed time, or plan such a time, for example go for a walk together.

- **The right issue**. The issue needs be something that the other person can change. For example, asking for your dad to lose 3 stone and stop smoking immediately is not realistic. Instead, discuss your concerns for his health and say how you're prepared to help him change to cut down smoking if he wants to.

- **The right words**. Use the approaches described in this workbook ('Broken record' and 'Saying no'). These techniques will help you to say what you need.

 Task

Think about how you can be more assertive in your own life. If you recognise that you lack assertiveness, try to:

- Use one of the assertiveness techniques during the next week.

- Remind yourself about and put into practice the **rules of assertiveness**. Copy page **223** or tear it out and carry it around with you. Put is somewhere you will see it (for example by your television or on a door or mirror or on the fridge) to remind you of these rules.

 Credit-card-sized versions of the rules of assertiveness and the seven steps of problem solving are available for you to print or order from **www.fiveareas.com**.

My notes

Overcoming Teenage Low Mood and Depression

A Five Areas Approach

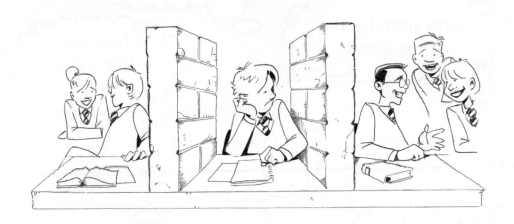

Building relationships

Helping you to help yourself
www.livinglifetothefull.com
www.fiveareas.com

Dr Nicky Dummett and Dr Chris Williams

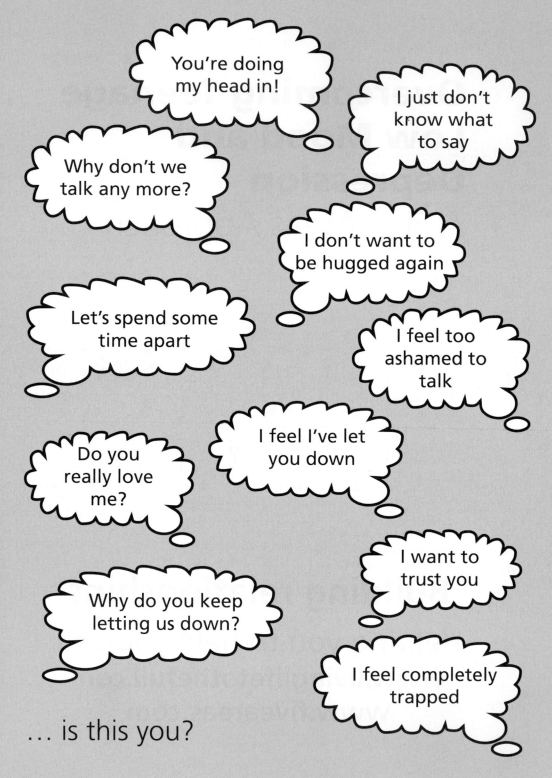

... is this you?

If it is ... this **workbook is for you**.

In this workbook you will:

- Review your style of communicating with others
- Learn how to build (and rebuild) close relationships.

Building relationships

We are all different. Some of us have many friends and acquaintances. Others prefer to keep themselves to themselves and have fewer people around who are 'close' to them. Whatever kind of relationship you prefer, it can be affected during times of upset.

Our past and present relationships are some of the most powerful things that affect how we feel. The relationships we have in our childhood influence how we relate to others in other ways too. For example, if parents are away a lot, or if we feel they've let us down, we may grow to mistrust others who actually can be trusted in future. Our relationships in childhood also teach us different ways or styles of relating to people and then we relate to others in the similar ways too.

Thus, our upbringing teaches us rules about:

- How we should communicate with others – with assertiveness, passivity or aggression (these terms are explained in the *Being assertive* workbook)
- How we expect others to relate to us – whether we can trust them or whether we think they will let us down.

Some of the rules are helpful and positive – for example, that we are loved, trusted and accepted. But sometimes the rules we learn are more negative and unhelpful.

Most of us learn a mixture of both helpful and unhelpful rules in childhood and these can affect how we react to others – especially when we're upset.

 Task

Use the checklist below to find out about your own helpful and unhelpful styles of relating.

'Rules' for our relationships that we have learnt from past experience	How this affects our relationships now (our relationship style)	Tick here if this applies to you – even if only sometimes
We may learn mostly positive things about how we see ourselves, others and our relationships. We have a reasonable self-esteem – that is, we feel good about ourselves	We mostly like who we are and so have good self-esteem. We usually think well of others while realising that we and they have faults. We trust others, and make a commitment in relationships. This is a healthy state to be in and one to aim for	☐
We may develop a low sense of worth or self-esteem. For example, we doubt whether we can be loved. We may believe we are ugly, boring or not worthy of being loved. We may think that if others knew the 'real' us they would run a mile	We put on a front and can't be ourselves. We can end up being clingy and dependent in our relationships. And we passively do anything to keep people happy (see the *Being assertive* workbook). We may use alcohol or drugs because we think they make us more 'interesting'	☐
We develop the opposite of the above rule – that is, high but fragile self-esteem that is linked to an inner neediness where we crave to be loved or needed. We may have been taught as a child that the whole world revolves around us. We see ourselves as special. If there are problems, we think these are caused by others	We can be very demanding of others. Things must revolve around us. We need to get our own way. We're often impatient with others who don't 'see the point'. We may seek out passive friends who will look up to us and do what we want. At the same time we may know we could always do better. Being in charge really matters. Yet you may quickly feel dissatisfied with what you do and also with people and want to move on	☐
We think of ourselves as ugly or not worthy of being loved	We may feel uncomfortable and avoid forming close relationships and commitment to protect ourselves from hurt ('It will never last'). We may dress down and hide our good points by wearing looser clothes. We may give up and 'let ourselves go'. Or we may become obsessed with looking 'just right'. We may flirt to test out whether we're really attractive. Or we may constantly test the love of those who care for us	☐

'Rules' for our relationships that we have learnt from past experience	How this affects our relationships now (our relationship style)	Tick here if this applies to you – even if only sometimes
Sometimes things that have happened in our life may teach us rules that show others aren't to be trusted. We may have learned that people we love will let us down or abandon us	We may find it hard to commit or respond with trust to others – even when they want to make a commitment to us. Our lack of trust may end up driving them away	☐
Sometimes our doubts can lead to jealous worries or anger	Jealousy comes from fear and can badly damage our relationships. We may make demands that our friends commit themselves to us	☐
I must not show my feelings. You may have learnt it's dangerous to show your feelings, or that being seen to be upset is a sign of weakness	You may have often heard that its typical of boys and men to bottle up their feelings. They rely on drink or work to block how they feel. Girls and women may be happier discussing their feelings and relationships with others. But of course boys or girls can behave either way. What matters more is the match (or mismatch) between two people. For example, when one person feels distressed and is struggling to cope, they may desperately want to discuss their problem with their family or a close friend. But the friend or family may not want to or feel able to. This clash can lead to more problems for the first person	☐

Think about where you learnt these helpful and unhelpful behaviours. Many people think that when they have a problem, the fault must be with themselves rather than the rules by which they have lived with all their life. This is because the rules may have worked in their home, but they don't work when they are in other places where others react in different ways.

The good news is that when this happens, we can look back and see things as they are.

Key point

People often have depression when they blame themselves for their failures and problems rather than realising it may simply be the time to see if their rules for relating to others are really suited to their present life.

Repeating behaviours in relationships

The rules we've learnt about in the workbook can explain why sometimes we repeat the same behaviours in friendships over and over again. Sometimes this works well, but sometimes we may end up repeating the same mistakes again and again.

For example, do you find yourself seeking out or being attracted to people who will hurt you in some way – that is, ignore your needs or put you down, or control you?

Another good question to ask about your close friendships is 'Do I feel I can be myself in this relationship?'

Our repeating behaviours can help us understand why we always go for the same kind of person and why we sometimes keep making the same mistakes. Becoming aware of these repeated behaviours is the first step towards changing them. And then we can learn new rules.

Remember you need to be aware of the rules and beliefs you have about you, your family, friends and relatives. They will affect how you relate and behave with others.

How do you relate to people you are close to?

The following questions will help you to think about your attitudes and reactions towards the people you are close to, for example your family and close friends. You may be tempted to answer these questions quite quickly with what you think to be the 'correct' answer.

Remember as you go through the questions, you'll get the most from this if you really think hard about the questions. The idea isn't to make you feel bad about yourself. Instead this will help you to begin to think about things that you may need to change for you to build more enjoyable relationships.

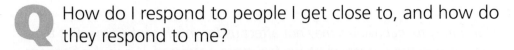

Q How do I respond to people I get close to, and how do they respond to me?

Think back on your present and past close relationships.

Q What **helpful** relationship styles do you repeat?

Q What **unhelpful** relationship styles do you repeat?

Q How do these repeated behaviours affect your relationships – now and in the past?

Q How do you think these behaviours affect how you respond when you feel distressed (for example suddenly ending a relationship when there are upsets, or always giving way)?

Q Do you often feel uncomfortable when speaking about how you or the people you're close to feel (for example some people find it hard to say sorry, or to offer a different opinion even about everyday things)?

Q Do you try to avoid speaking about how you feel? How do those around you react to this?

Our unhelpful behaviours may not affect us for much of the time. But they can come to the surface when we feel more distressed. When this happens they can unhelpfully disrupt how we react to those who we are close to.

Things you can do that can make a difference

Here are some things you could do and not do, to build friendships and relationships.

With people you don't know so well
Do

- Be yourself.

- Plan a short answer to respond with if someone asks 'How are you?' Remember, they don't know you well. They may well not be aware you are finding things hard at the moment. Don't feel you have to tell the person everything about yourself. Say something like 'Getting on fine thanks. How are you? Great weather isn't it?' And leave it at that.

Don't
- Tell everyone about every thing about your life and how you feel – try to remember that everyone you know isn't your friend.

With friends and family members you trust

Our wider family and friends can be a great support for us. One of the workbooks in this book, called *Ideas for families and friends: how can I offer the best support?*, is for them. You might wish to show this workbook to them or even plan to go through it together. You may also get some thoughts from this workbook yourself that you can share with them.

Do
- Try to get support from close friends.

- Try out new things to help you learn about yourself and your relationships. But make sure you try one small change at time – people and relationships take time to change.

- Try to keep in mind the other person's feelings as well. They may also have reasons for emotions such as anger, jealousy, anxiety and upset. You need to work out what these reasons are and slowly tackle them together. Be aware how these things affect both your friendships and your romantic relationships. For example, are you using your old rules of unhelpful thinking?

- Learn how to still have a good relationship with someone even when you disagree.

- Keep lines of communication open – even when you don't feel like it.

- Make time to be together, setting aside any problems for a while. Sometimes this can help free you both up to be different.

- Ask yourself whether you are avoiding each other, or avoiding discussing the real problems. Bear in mind that sometimes the other person may not be ready to make changes.

Don't
- Become dependent on others or think that only they can help.

- Become overly involved in just one friendship.

- Mistake friendship for romance.

Rebuilding your relationships by building communication and commitment

Many young people have relationships that they can't easily change, for example some family relationships that have been there for a long time. So, we may need to be realistic about what can and what can't change.

What you can change is:

- What life rules **you** use in different areas of your life

- What relationships you choose for the future.

Remember, we don't know if we can change things unless we try. A key question is how much improvement you and the other person both feel you need to make to improve things. At the same time we don't want to be overly hard on ourselves – feeling we have failed if others are unwilling to change.

Sometimes you may need to make only **some small changes** to improve your relationship. For example:

- **Listening**. Pay attention and don't just switch off and think you know what is being said. Talk about each other's day. Ask questions about the small but important things in your life.

- **Doing things together**. Spend time together going for walks, eating meals together, etc.

- **Tackling 'relationship killers'** – such as only doing things apart.

- **Trying to forgive each other.** Living with anger and guilt can eat away at a relationship. You may need to forgive each other – or ask for forgiveness from the other person if you've done things that have caused hurt. The first step will always be simply to let the other person know how you have felt and listen to them. Sometimes this is all you can do, and it may not make you feel any better immediately. **But it does mean that you have openly discussed things**. Sometimes, this can be all that you need to do because just knowing the other person has heard your side is helpful.

- **Bringing positives back into what you do**. Take any opportunity to say thank you, or to let someone know when they have made you feel good. Letting people know that they matter is far more important than buying an expensive gift.

Hearing what we expect to hear

The reason for many relationship problems is that the people don't communicate with each other. When we're distressed we tend to think about things in quite extreme and unhelpful ways. **This can have a big effect on how two people interpret the same conversation**. We may think that because we know each other so well, we already know what is going to be said. The trouble is that sometimes we can be wrong.

The problem is that **we don't actually listen to what the other person is really saying**. For example, we may say something like 'That was a nice meal' to our parent and mean it as a compliment. But because of hurt and upset our parent may hear it as 'Well you've cooked something nice for once – usually you don't make much effort'. The danger is that all kinds of positive replies can be taken in a negative way.

What should you do if this happens with you?

First, try to see it as a problem. You can do this by choosing to check out what the other person means. This will help you to avoid jumping to conclusions about each other. Remember to ask politely rather than in an angry or defensive way.

Try to stop yourself from reacting immediately when you think you've been hurt or insult. Check out what the other person meant rather than jumping to conclusions. If they really are trying to be critical this will quickly come out. But often you will find that you've simply misunderstood each other.

Violence and abuse

If you are being abused

Sadly, some young people are in bad relationships that they can't change. They may even be abused. They don't know that there are adults they can go to for support. **If you are being threatened or hit or touched sexually in a way that is not 'right' you should tell someone.** Sometimes it can be hard to choose who to trust, and you may be scared to tell anyone. Here are some ways you can get help:

- Contact ChildLine. The telephone number is 0800 1111 or you can visit the website (**www.childline.org.uk**).
- Tell a teacher you can trust.
- Talk to a close family member you can trust.
- Talk to an older friend you can trust.
- Talk to your doctor.
- Look again at the 'How do I know if I need extra help?' section in the *Understanding why I feel as I do* workbook.

You may not be aware that teachers, doctors and social workers have training in how best to help young people who need extra help.

If someone you know is being abused

Maybe you know of someone else who is close to you who is suffering violence or abuse. Again, you may be able to find someone like the people we've listed above who can help.

If you yourself are hitting, harming or abusing others

If you have been hitting, harming or abusing someone else, then you need to understand that this behaviour isn't right. It's called **bullying** others. Sometimes this may be new behaviour for you. You may have started doing this because of the anger you feel linked to your depression or tension. Or it may be because of something else that is going on in your life and is even being worsened by you drinking or taking drugs. Or it may be that violence and threats are something that you have done for a long time and in many of your relationships.

Do you think this is this a helpful way of dealing with relationships in your life? Please seek help using the suggestions we've given above or talk to your doctor. Your doctor can help without you being afraid of how they may react.

Summary

In this workbook you have:

- Learnt about your own style of communicating with others
- Learnt about how to build (and rebuild) relationships.

Let's look at the whole picture again

After you have been putting this workbook into action in your life for a while, rate the size of your problems again in each of the **five areas**.

Q Overall, do I have (or have I had) problems in Area 1: People and events?

No problems at all   The worst they could possibly be

0   5   10

Q Overall, do I have problems in Area 2: Altered thinking?

No problems at all   The worst they could possibly be

0   5   10

Q Overall, do I have problems in Area 3: Altered feelings?

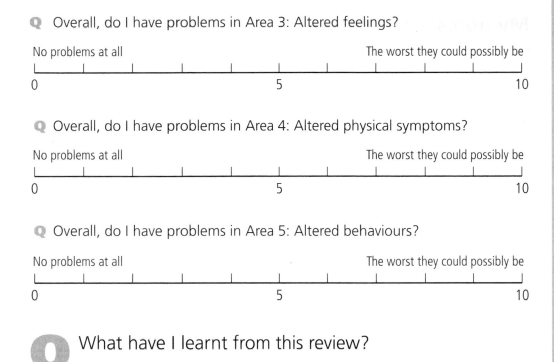

No problems at all   The worst they could possibly be

0   5   10

Q Overall, do I have problems in Area 4: Altered physical symptoms?

No problems at all   The worst they could possibly be

0   5   10

Q Overall, do I have problems in Area 5: Altered behaviours?

No problems at all   The worst they could possibly be

0   5   10

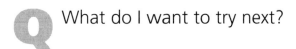 What have I learnt from this review?

Q What do I want to try next?

Putting into practice what you have learnt

Is there anyone you want to show this workbook to? Think about reading it through together. You might want to go through the *Ideas for families and friends* workbook as well.

A Five Areas assessment of sleeplessness

Many things can affect our sleep and these are described below. Think about whether they affect your life.

Area 1: People and events
Your physical environment

● Is your bed comfortable?

● What about the temperature of the room where you sleep? If the room is either very cold or very hot this might make it hard to go to sleep.

● Is the room very noisy?

● Is there too much light in the room? If bright lights such as streetlights come through your curtains, this can also prevent you sleeping.

Q Do I try to sleep in a poor sleep environment?

Yes ☐   No ☐

If you answered 'Yes', you could try looking at some of these things to help you sleep better.

Poor mattress
If your mattress is quite old, can you turn it over, rotate it or even change it? Can you add extra support, such as a board or old door underneath it?

Too hot or too cold
If it is too hot, try opening a window or using a fan. If it is too cold, think about using an extra blanket or duvet. Or you could think about insulation, draught excluders or secondary or double-glazing. (You will need to speak to the adults responsible for the house to see if any of these are possible.)

Problems with noise
Reduce the noise around you if you can. Can someone speak to noisy brothers, sisters or neighbours to ask them to turn down their television or music? Have you or any one in your family thought about fitting double glazing or internal plastic sheeting over windows to reduce noise? This needn't be expensive and many reasonably priced options are available.

Problems with excessive light
Consider the thickness of your curtains. Have you or any family members thought about adding a thicker lining or blackout lining? If this may not be

possible, for example because of the cost involved, a black plastic bin bag can work well as a blackout blind. It can be stapled or stuck to the curtain rail.

Area 2: Altered thinking

Anxious thoughts are a common cause of sleeplessness. You may have anxious thoughts about your life in general, or you may worry about not sleeping.

- You may worry that you will not be able to sleep at all.
- You may worry that sleeplessness will reduce your ability to concentrate the next day.
- Your fears get blown out of proportion and prevent you going off to sleep.
- Another common fear is that your brain or your body will be harmed by lack of sleep.

In sleep, your tension levels go down, so your body and brain begin to relax. In contrast, when you're anxious, your brain becomes overly alert. You end up mulling over things again and again. This is the exact opposite of what's needed to go to sleep. Worrying thoughts are therefore both a cause and an effect of poor sleep.

Q Do I worry about things in general?

Yes ☐   No ☐

Task

If you answered 'Yes', Read the *Noticing and changing extreme and unhelpful thinking* workbook.

Q Do I worry about not sleeping?

Yes ☐   No ☐

If you answered 'Yes', write down your worries on a notepad. You will need to challenge any extreme fears about the consequences of not sleeping. Studies show that most people do not need very much sleep at all to be physically and mentally healthy. When people who may have poor sleep are asked to try to sleep in a sleep research laboratory, many actually sleep far more than they think. Sometimes people who are in a light level of sleep dream that they are awake. You therefore may be sleeping more than you think.

You also need to know that not sleeping enough doesn't have a very big effect on your brain or your body. It is possible to still function with very little sleep each night.

Q Do I have extreme fears about the consequences of not sleeping?

Yes ☐   No ☐

Extreme (catastrophic) fears can themselves cause increased wakefulness, thus preventing you going off to sleep. It is important for you to know that these thoughts are extreme, inaccurate and unhelpful. Although you might feel tired and irritable, this doesn't necessarily affect your ability to do things around the house or at school.

📌 **Task**

If worrying thoughts are a problem for you, read the *Noticing and changing extreme and unhelpful thinking* workbook.

Area 3: Altered physical problems

Pain, itching or other physical symptoms can cause sleeplessness. Tackling these physical symptoms will help with your sleep problems.

Q Are physical symptoms keeping me awake?

Yes ☐   No ☐

If you answered 'Yes', please see your doctor to get the right medical treatment for your symptoms. Sometimes if you have depression or anxiety, your physical symptoms can feel worse. Your doctor then may offer you treatment for your low mood or anxious mood to help reduce the physical symptoms.

Area 4: Altered feelings

Many feelings can be linked to sleeplessness.

Q Do I feel anxious when I try to sleep?

Yes ☐   No ☐

If you answered 'Yes', remember that anxiety is a common cause of sleeplessness. It often triggers your body's fear response, causing adrenaline to flow. This causes you to feel fidgety or restless. You may notice physical symptoms such as an increase in your heart rate and breathing rate, a churning feeling in your stomach or tension throughout your body. Your anxiety therefore acts to keep you alert. This is the opposite of what you want to be when you're trying to fall off to sleep. Sometimes we may become anxious about sleeping (for example if we have nightmares or wake up feeling panicky).

Q Am I feeling depressed, upset or low in mood and do I no longer enjoy things as before?

Yes ☐   No ☐

If you answered 'Yes', remember that depression is a common cause of sleeplessness. For example, when we are feeling depressed we may find that it takes us up to several hours to get off to sleep. We may wake up several hours earlier than normal feeling we haven't rested or feeling on edge. Having treatment for our depression can often be helpful for improving our sleep.

Other emotions such as shame, guilt and anger can also cause sleeplessness.

Area 5: Altered behaviour: unhelpful behaviours
Preparing for sleep

The time leading up to sleep is very important. Try to build in a '**wind-down**' time in the evening when you are less active and engaged in less stimulating activity. Physical over-activity such as exercising, eating too much, playing computer games or watching television just before going to bed can keep you awake. Sometimes people watch television while lying in bed. This may help them wind down, but many people become more alert and so it adds to their sleep problems.

Q Am I doing things which wake me up when I should be winding down?

Yes ☐   No ☐

If you answered 'Yes', keep your bed as a place for sleep. Don't lie on your bed watching television, working or worrying. This will only wake you up and prevent you sleeping. You'll also need to decide whether listening to a radio or music helps you go to sleep.

Q Overall, do I have problems in Area 5: Altered behaviours?

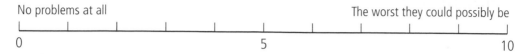

No problems at all   The worst they could possibly be

0   5   10

 What have I learnt from this review?

 What do I want to try next?

Putting into practice what you have learnt

Look back at the **sleep checklists of things to do and not do** on pages 256–8. Plan to make changes in how you prepare for sleep and what you do once you are in bed.

Write down what you're going to do this week to put into practice what you have learnt.

My practice plan

Q What changes am I going to make?

Q When am I going to do it?

Q What problems could arise, and how can I sort these?

Apply the **questions for effective change** to your plan.

Q Is my planned task one that:

- Will be useful for understanding or changing how I am?

Yes ☐ No ☐

- Is a specific task so that I will know when I have done it?

Yes ☐ No ☐

3 Socially (on you and others)

● **Longer term** (look back to over the past 6 to 12 months)

1 Physically

2 Psychologically

3 Socially (on you and others)

If after reading this workbook you have discovered that your drinking or drug use is causing harm to you or others, then **you need to tackle it**.

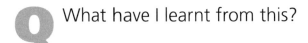 What have I learnt from this?

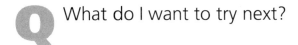 What do I want to try next?

How to make changes

Try to reduce your overall intake of alcohol or drugs each week. If possible, build in at least **two days** without any drink or drugs to allow your body to recover.

If you're drinking or using street drugs at a far higher level

If you stop drinking or taking the drugs too quickly, you may notice some symptoms of withdrawal. This is probably the reason why so many people fail to tackle this problem. But it's possible to make changes – and it's even more important to do so if you're having a lot of drinks or drugs. (See page **267** for the recommended amounts of drinks for men and women.)

To change yourself successfully you need to cut down the amount you're taking in a **slow step-by-step manner** You may find the *Unhelpful things we do* workbook useful for some ideas of how to plan this. But if you're taking drugs or drinking alcohol at higher levels, it's best to make these changes together with some help and advice from your general practitioner (GP), local drug or alcohol support services or other healthcare practitioner.

> *If you regularly use street drugs or drink excessive alcohol, please* **discuss** *this with someone who can help*. *If you are doing these things on a regular basis, it may prevent you getting better.*

Other ways to get help

Look at your local *Yellow Pages*, and also the following national organisations:

- NHS Direct (England and Wales). This will provide you with help and advice on any aspect of drug and alcohol use. Tel. 0845 4647; website **www.nhsdirect.nhs.uk**

- NHS24 (Scotland). This is the equivalent site for Scotland for advice and assessment. Tel. 08454 24242; website: **www.nhs24.com**

- Royal College of Psychiatrists. The College has an information sheet about drugs and alcohol. It includes many useful links. Visit the website: **www.rcpsych.ac.uk/mentalhealthinformation/mentalhealthand growingup/36drugsandalcohol.aspx**

- Talk to Frank. This website has stories, information and resources about drugs, including information for the person taking drugs and also for their family and friends. You can talk on the phone and ask for information from a counsellor or you can e-mail or access the help online, including Franks Infobus (set times only – see website). Tel. 0800 776600; website: **www.talktofrank.com** (Please note: Frank is **not** a real person but the website acts as a way for you to get straight advice and info about drugs. It gives you the facts without the attitude.)

Summary

In this workbook you have:

- Learnt some useful facts about alcohol and street drugs

- Learnt how alcohol and street drugs can mess people up

- Learnt how you can work out what effects they're having on you

- Learnt how to plan some next steps to bring about change if you have a problem.

Let's look at the whole picture again

After you have been putting this workbook into action in your life for a while, rate the size of your problems again in each of the **five areas**.

Q Overall, do I have (or have I had) problems in Area 1: People and events?

No problems at all .... The worst they could possibly be

0   5   10

Q Overall, do I have problems in Area 2: Altered thinking?

No problems at all .... The worst they could possibly be

0   5   10

Q Overall, do I have problems in Area 3: Altered feelings?

No problems at all .... The worst they could possibly be

0   5   10

Q Overall, do I have problems in Area 4: Altered physical symptoms?

No problems at all   The worst they could possibly be

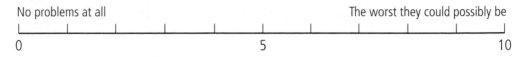

0   5   10

Q Overall, do I have problems in Area 5: Altered behaviours?

No problems at all   The worst they could possibly be

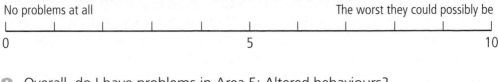

0   5   10

Q What have I learnt from this review?

Q What do I want to try next?

Putting into practice what you have learnt

Write down any action points you need to do this week. Do you need to ask anyone any questions? Is there anything else you need to do?

My practice plan

Q What changes am I going to make?

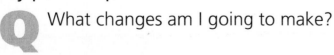

My notes

Drink and street drug diary: my week

Day and date	Morning	Afternoon	Evening	Total units or cost
Monday				Total units/day = Cost/day £
Tuesday				Total units/day = Cost/day £
Wednesday				Total units/day = Cost/day £
Thursday				Total units/day = Cost/day £
Friday				Total units/day = Cost/day £
Saturday				Total units/day = Cost/day £
Sunday				Total units/day = Cost/day £
			Weekly total	

Remember to record everything you drink/take.

Overcoming Teenage Low Mood and Depression

A Five Areas Approach

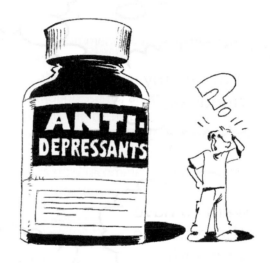

Understanding and using anti-depressant medication

Helping you to help yourself
www.livinglifetothefull.com
www.fiveareas.com

Dr Nicky Dummett and Dr Chris Williams

Some other times when anti-depressants may be used

Other than for depression, anti-depressants are also **sometimes** used to treat a variety of mental and physical health problems. These include:

- Anxiety and tension
- Panic attacks
- Physical symptoms such as chronic fatigue and pain.

It's important to understand from your doctor the reason why you may be prescribed an anti-depressant.

Frequently asked questions

 Why do we use anti-depressant medication for the treatment of depression?

Remember the Five Areas model: there are links between the altered thinking, feelings, behaviour and physical aspects of depression. Because of the links between each of the areas, the **physical treatment** offered by medication can lead to positive improvements in the other areas too.

The Five Areas assessment model

Life situations, relationships, practical problems

Medication works here

Altered thinking

Altered feelings

Altered physical symptoms

Altered behaviour

How well do anti-depressant tablets work?

Anti-depressant medication can help lift symptoms in moderate or severe depression in about two-thirds of young people. Usually you get the best out of them when you're also having a talking treatment such as cognitive behaviour therapy or family therapy at the same time.

How long do they take to work?

Do not expect immediate results. Anti-depressant medicines take about two to four weeks to begin to work and their positive effects may take up to four to six weeks to happen. Most people notice a substantial improvement in how they feel after two to four weeks of starting an anti-depressant medicine.

Therefore it's very important that you take the tablets regularly and for long enough, even if to begin with they seem like they aren't working. Sometimes, doctors tell you to take a smaller dose of the anti-depressant medicine to start with but then they may slowly increase the dose over a number of weeks or months if this is needed.

Key point

You shouldn't give up on your anti-depressant medicine if you don't notice changes straight away.

Do anti-depressants have side effects?

All tablets have side effects. The important question is whether the side effects of having untreated depression are worse. The modern anti-depressant medicines recommended for use in young people usually have few side effects. For example, they usually don't cause drowsiness.

Many side effects disappear within a few days of starting the tablets as you get used to them. Sometimes anxiety can actually worsen how much we notice our symptoms. Your doctor should have gone through the possible side effects with you when you started treatment. But you can ask them again if you are unsure, and you can read the manufacturer's information leaflet.

This is because of the particular way in which anti-depressants work. It means they will not help you feel better at the time you take the higher dose anyway.

*Misusing tablets by taking more than what your doctor has told you to take can backfire and worsen the way you feel. This is because taking tablets at higher than recommended doses may cause you to have side effects. It may also be **unhelpful** because it wrongly teaches you that you're only managing to cope because of using the medication. You then come to believe that you can't live life without the tablets.*

Stopping anti-depressants

Sometimes we may be tempted to stop taking medication without telling our doctor. We may be afraid we are letting them down, or that we will be 'told off' if we do. It is actually better to discuss any worries you have openly with your doctor. It is also important when stopping anti-depressants to do this gradually by making a timetable with your doctor. Otherwise, you may get withdrawal symptoms.

***Stopping an anti-depressant too early is the commonest cause of worsening depression**. The national guidelines advise doctors to tell their patients to continue to take the anti-depressant medication for at least six months after feeling better to prevent slipping back into depression.*

Putting things into practice

If you want to find out more about the use of anti-depressant medications please discuss this with your doctor. They will be able to suggest other sources of information about the treatments that are available.

Summary

In this workbook you have:

- Learnt how anti-depressants are used

- Found out the answers to some common questions

- Learnt some useful hints and tips to get the best out of medication

- Learnt about the pluses and minuses of medication if this is being suggested for you.

Let's look at the whole picture again

If you have been prescribed anti-depressant medication, after you have been using them for at least six weeks, rate the size of your problems again in each of the **five areas**.

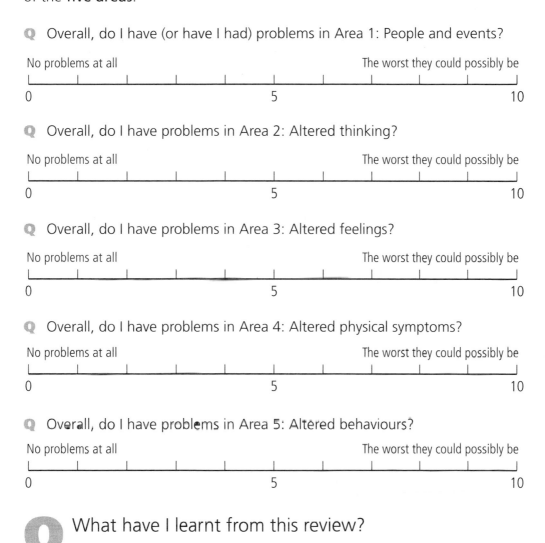

Q Overall, do I have (or have I had) problems in Area 1: People and events?

No problems at all   The worst they could possibly be

0   5   10

Q Overall, do I have problems in Area 2: Altered thinking?

No problems at all   The worst they could possibly be

0   5   10

Q Overall, do I have problems in Area 3: Altered feelings?

No problems at all   The worst they could possibly be

0   5   10

Q Overall, do I have problems in Area 4: Altered physical symptoms?

No problems at all   The worst they could possibly be

0   5   10

Q Overall, do I have problems in Area 5: Altered behaviours?

No problems at all   The worst they could possibly be

0   5   10

Q What have I learnt from this review?

Q What do I want to try next?

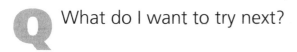

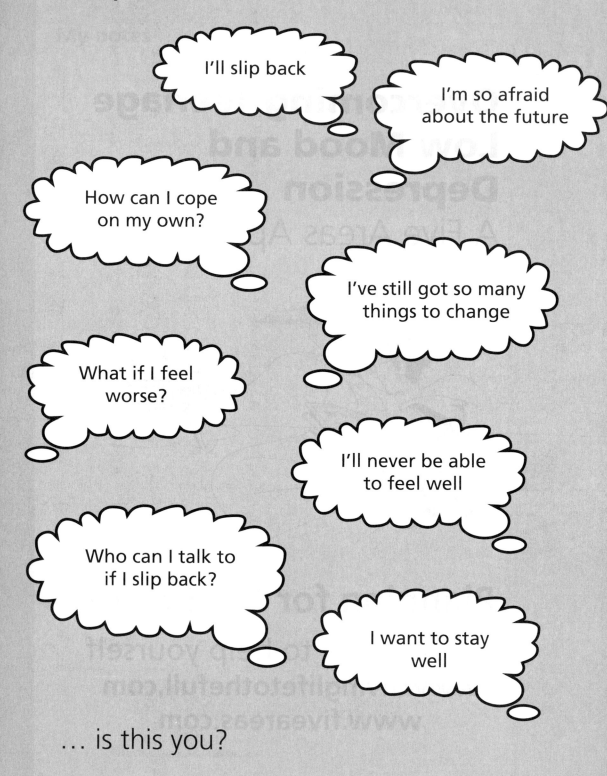

… is this you?

If it is … this **workbook is for you**.

In this workbook you will:

- Have a chance to look back at what you have learned

- Summarise key lessons you have learned

- Work out 'danger signs' that things may be slipping back

- Develop a clear plan to stay well

- Set up some review days so you can check your own progress.

The journey of recovery

It can sometimes be helpful to think of yourself as being on a **journey of recovery**. When you first started working on your problems, you probably had lots of different problems you wished to tackle.

By using the course workbooks we hope things have improved in at least some areas since you began your journey down this path. In the following sections there are some questions to help you identify **what has been helpful for you** and what things have helped you move on.

My journey

 Task

 What is different now from before?

 What gains have I made?

Other Five Areas material that you can use includes:

- *Overcoming Anxiety: A Five Areas Approach* by Dr Chris Williams (2003). Hodder Arnold: London. This book focuses on generalised anxiety or worry, panic and phobias, obsessive–compulsive disorder (OCD) materials and anxiety in physical health problems.

- **www.fiveareas.com**: the central resource area to access all Five Areas material.

A request for feedback

The content of this workbook is updated and improved on a regular basis based on feedback from users and practitioners. If there are areas in the workbook that you found hard to understand, or that seemed unclear please let us know. However, we don't to provide any specific advice on treatment.

To provide feedback please contact us:

- Via our website: **www.livinglifetothefull.com**. Register and use the 'Contact Us' link at the top of the homepage.

- Or by e-mail: **feedback@fiveareas.com**. In your feedback, please can you state which workbook or book you are referring to.

My notes

PART 3

Support materials for relatives and friends

Overcoming Teenage Low Mood and Depression

A Five Areas Approach

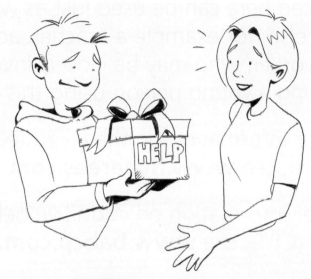

Ideas for families and friends: how can I offer the best support?

Helping you to help yourself
www.livinglifetothefull.com
www.fiveareas.com

Dr Nicky Dummett and Dr Chris Williams

This workbook is aimed at those important family members and friends who may be able to support a young person with low mood. It summarises the key elements of the Five Areas course so that you can understand how it works and offer support in the best possible way.

Although this workbook mainly talks about family and friends, the general points and skills introduced here can be used just as well by anyone else, for example a teacher, advisor or youth worker, who may be closely involved in supporting a young person using this approach.

For other information on the Five Areas Approach, see **www.fiveareas.com**.

For other information on cognitive behaviour therapy (CBT), see **www.babcp.com**.

To view the Living Life to the Full course, please sign up at **www.livinglifetothefull.com**.

In this workbook you will:

- Learn what happens when a young person has low mood or depression
- Understand what this course is about – and how the young person is using it
- Learn helpful and unhelpful responses
- Learn ways to offer support that will help and ways to communicate more clearly
- Learn ways to look after ourselves and stay well
- Learn when extra help is needed and where to go for it.

The Five Areas Approach

The course workbooks use a proven approach that is based on cognitive behaviour therapy (CBT for short). CBT is a kind of 'talking treatment' that works well for people with low mood. It's recommended by the latest UK national treatment guidelines for young people with low mood and depression.

These workbooks help us look in detail at five key areas of our life. The aim is to help the young person to do a **Five Areas Assessment**. This assessment clearly shows the person the range of problems we may face in each of the five areas that are commonly affected in low mood and depression:

- Area 1: People and events around us
- Area 2: Altered thinking
- Area 3: Altered feelings (also called moods or emotions)
- Area 4: Altered physical symptoms in our body
- Area 5: Altered behaviour or activity levels. (This includes both helpful and unhelpful things we do that can make us feel better or backfire on how we feel.)

  *The areas are all **linked**. So what happens in any one area can cause changes in other areas. For example, what we **think** about a situation or problem affects how we feel **emotionally and physically** and also affects what we do. How we feel affects what we **think** (for example seeing just the down side of things).*

When we have a low mood or we have depression, **vicious circles** happen that worsen things and keep our problems going. A Five Areas Assessment can show us how this is happening. For example:

Ian's Five Areas assessment

Area 1: People and events
- Bullying at school
- Dropped from a sports team
- Gran died two years ago

Area 2: Altered thinking
- Focuses on how things have gone wrong and that things will get worse and that it is all his fault
- Things seem pointless or too difficult, for example having fun and talking to people
- Thinks that he has failed repeatedly
- Worries about what other people will think
- Doesn't notice when the things he is worried about don't actually happen

Area 3: Altered feelings
Starts to feel down, anxious and guilty

Area 4: Altered physical symptoms
- Low energy and tiredness
- Poor concentration
- Even everyday things are harder than usual

Area 5: Altered behaviour
- Reduced activity levels, especially things that usually make him feel better through a sense of pleasure, achievement or closeness to others
- Avoids social contact
- Turns inwards – doesn't talk about even day-to-day experiences, let alone things that are more difficult to talk about
- Tries out fewer new things and puts off or ignores problems
- Sets himself up to fail in ways that 'confirm' his failure
- Lashes out or tries to block how he feels, for example verbal or physical aggression or alcohol or drug misuse
- Tests out relationships with risky or provocative behaviour
- Avoids specific situations, people or events that seem scary so his life becomes even more stressful

The result is a vicious circle that just goes round and round. To find out if this vicious circle is happening for the person you know, read on.

The **first** causes of low mood are very often mainly outside the young person. In other words, the causes are often first from things in **Area 1: People and events**. For example:

- Facing overwhelming stresses or challenges

- Long-standing family tensions

- Suffering loss (such as death of a loved one)

- Other long-term problems (such as illness)

- Long-standing lack of emotional support or insecurity in relationships

- Feeling powerless to change a situation around them.

Sometimes, the young person may not be getting the attention or support they need from those around them. This may be because for whatever reason their needs tend to be overlooked in the family or sometimes their basic needs are actually being **neglected**.

Some young people may even be suffering emotional, physical or sexual **abuse**. As a family member or friend, you may be best placed to recognise this and help them find appropriate help, possibly from social services, their general practitioner (GP) or other support services.

 Think of the young person you know who has low mood or depression. If they carried out a **life review** of their Area 1 by answering the questions below, would it show that they have any particular problems?

Importantly, do other people need to make changes too?

While some things listed below can be a positive change at the right time in a young person's life (for example getting their own place), is the change something they have actually **chosen** to do and something that is helpful **now**?

Family and home: Does this cause problems for me?

1 I have problems getting on with one or more of my parents or carers.

Often ☐   Sometimes ☐   No ☐

2 I have problems getting on with another person or people in my family.

Often ☐   Sometimes ☐   No ☐

3 Other people in my family don't get on.

Often ☐   Sometimes ☐   No ☐

4 One or both of my parents or carers has been absent, left home or gone away.

Often ☐   Sometimes ☐   No ☐

5 I am now living separately from some or all of my family.

Often ☐   Sometimes ☐   No ☐

6 My family has housing problems (for example too small or may have to leave).

Often ☐   Sometimes ☐   No ☐

7 My family has unemployment (joblessness) or money worries.

Often ☐   Sometimes ☐   No ☐

8 I am or we are having problems with neighbours.

Often ☐   Sometimes ☐   No ☐

Friends and other relationships

9 I've fallen out with one or more of my friends.

Often ☐   Sometimes ☐   No ☐

10 There is no-one around that I can really talk to.

Often ☐   Sometimes ☐   No ☐

11 A person or people important to me has been out of contact or gone away.

Often ☐   Sometimes ☐   No ☐

Practical problems

12 I or someone else close to me has physical or mental health problems.

Often ☐　　　　Sometimes ☐　　　　No ☐

13 I or someone else close to me has drug or alcohol problems.

Often ☐　　　　Sometimes ☐　　　　No ☐

14 I or we face other practical problems at the moment.

Often ☐　　　　Sometimes ☐　　　　No ☐

School or college

15 I have problems with school or college work, exams or tests.

Often ☐　　　　Sometimes ☐　　　　No ☐

16 I have problems with attending or staying in school or college.

Often ☐　　　　Sometimes ☐　　　　No ☐

17 I have recently changed school or college.

Often ☐　　　　Sometimes ☐　　　　No ☐

18 I have problems with other people my age at school or college.

Often ☐　　　　Sometimes ☐　　　　No ☐

19 I have problems with staff at my school or college.

Often ☐　　　　Sometimes ☐　　　　No ☐

20 I am being bullied or picked on.

Often ☐　　　　Sometimes ☐　　　　No ☐

Things that have happened in my life: Are any still happening?

21 Someone has been doing or saying things they shouldn't so that I didn't or don't feel safe.

Often ☐　　　　Sometimes ☐　　　　No ☐

22 Something else has happened that has really upset or harmed me or someone close to me.

Often ☐　　　　Sometimes ☐　　　　No ☐

Write here any other problem(s) they may have. Also, write here any other information you have about any of the questions. Say which question number it is and when the problem happened. Is it still happening? Use an extra sheet of paper if you need (or use the My notes pages at the back of this workbook):

Now think about the other four areas of the young person's life.

Area 2: Altered thinking

 Has the young person you know:

- Been saying that things seem hopeless?

Yes ☐   No ☐   Sometimes ☐

- Been saying that things seem pointless or too hard?

Yes ☐   No ☐   Sometimes ☐

● Been able to see only the negative side of things?

Yes ☐　　　　No ☐　　　　Sometimes ☐

● Been blaming themselves unnecessarily?

Yes ☐　　　　No ☐　　　　Sometimes ☐

● Been spending a lot of time dwelling on things?

Yes ☐　　　　No ☐　　　　Sometimes ☐

Area 3: Altered feelings

Q Has the young person you know:

● Been overly anxious?

Yes ☐　　　　No ☐　　　　Sometimes ☐

● Been overly low in mood?

Yes ☐　　　　No ☐　　　　Sometimes ☐

● Been overly guilty about things?

Yes ☐　　　　No ☐　　　　Sometimes ☐

● Been overly angry/irritable about things?

Yes ☐　　　　No ☐　　　　Sometimes ☐

● Been feeling very embarrassed/ashamed about things?

Yes ☐　　　　No ☐　　　　Sometimes ☐

Area 4: Altered physical symptoms

Q Has the young person you know:

● Been feeling tired a lot, with poor energy?

Yes ☐　　　　No ☐　　　　Sometimes ☐

- Been off their food or losing weight or started to over-eat?

Yes ☐   No ☐   Sometimes ☐

Area 5: Altered behaviour

Q Has the young person you know:

- Reduced their overall activity levels a lot?

Yes ☐   No ☐   Sometimes ☐

- Stopped doing activities that bring pleasure, achievement or closeness?

Yes ☐   No ☐   Sometimes ☐

- Been avoiding social contact?

Yes ☐   No ☐   Sometimes ☐

- Been talking less about even everyday things?

Yes ☐   No ☐   Sometimes ☐

- Been doing a lot of unhelpful behaviours? (For example, risk taking, using drugs, isolating themselves)

Yes ☐   No ☐   Sometimes ☐

- Been testing out relationships with threats or risk taking?

Yes ☐   No ☐   Sometimes ☐

- Been avoiding situations or events and restricting their life?

Yes ☐   No ☐   Sometimes ☐

Write down anything else you have noticed here.

The good news is that making helpful changes in any one of the areas can lead to benefits in the others areas as well and help people recover. The workbooks in this course aim to help a young person to do just that.

About low mood and depression in young people

Low mood and depression in young people are **common**. There are nearly always several causes for low mood and depression. Once depression has got going, it can then either keep going on or go away depending on the way the young person reacts.

Sometimes the young person's responses can be helpful, and the vicious circle dies down and the person recovers. But at other times the altered thinking and behaviour spiral down and down and make things worse. For example, when a young person feels down or depressed they may try even harder than usual to meet unrealistic standards or goals they have set themselves (such as feeling they must always please other people). Usually these efforts don't work and the young person feels even more despondent about themselves.

Family and friends can provide real support, but some of their responses can also at times become part of the young person's problem. The Five Areas Approach helps both the young person and their family and friends to think **together** about which responses are helpful and which might be unhelpful.

About the course

The course is based on cognitive behaviour therapy (see page 315) and aims to help people bring about helpful changes in the five key areas of life. The course workbooks are practical and help us to stop, think and reflect on the impact of our thoughts and actions. They help us learn key skills that make a difference by breaking the vicious circles (like those described above). They also help us try out helpful behaviours and new ways of thinking.

The first steps involve working in **Area 5: Altered behaviour**. The young person is helped to gradually increase behaviours that help build positive mood by:

- Simply enjoying things around them, and so bringing **pleasure** to themselves and boosting their mood
- Bringing a sense of **achievement** and feeling good about themselves
- Bringing a sense of **closeness** to other people.

Overcoming Teenage Low Mood and Depression: A Five Areas Approach   © Dr Nicky Dummet and Dr Chris Williams (2008)

Making changes is something that needs to be done **gradually** at a pace and level the young person can cope with. It's important that they don't bite off more than they can chew at once. If they do this, they may not be able to make the helpful changes. Making changes takes time. You may need to help them be realistic and also help them overcome practical problems.

The course next helps the young person look at their thoughts that are upsetting them (**Area 2: Altered thinking**). The workbooks help them to think whether their thoughts are really 'true' or just based on a part of the picture (just looking at the negative side). They are encouraged to rediscover the 'bigger picture' by looking at the positive side too, to help them produce a more **balanced story** (taking into account all that's been happening, positive **and** negative). This approach also helps them to stop, think and reflect when they have similar thoughts in the future. Other workbooks deal with how to develop specific skills (for example learning to be assertive or learning how to solve problems) and overcome specific problems (for example sleep problems).

You can learn about the workbooks the young person is using by reading them yourself (they are listed in the *Understanding why I feel as I do* workbook). Many young people, quite reasonably, don't want to show others their actual answers to the questions in the workbooks, preferring to keep them to themselves. If so, you will need to respect their wishes and resist any temptation to read their notes without their permission. But the workbooks do encourage young people to find ways to share with close friends or family anything they need to discuss to move forward.

How family and friends can help

It can be confusing trying to work out how best to offer support. Sometimes, a **life review** (above) of **Area 1** makes it clear that other situations or relationships or people need to change **before** the young person can start to feel better. Also, it can be hard getting the **right balance** of offering support without becoming too protective and wrapping them in cotton wool. Sometimes, the young person may need to be encouraged to face up to challenges, but remember to do this at a pace they can cope with. Usually, **extremes of response** (for example extreme over-protection or extreme under-protection) are likely to be unhelpful, but occasionally they may be the right things to do just for a short time.

Example: Being too protective

Ian has become depressed and can't concentrate well. For a long time, Mum made excuses for him about doing any homework tasks, which took the pressure off Ian. But this also meant that he didn't get the chance to do the easier homework that he could've still done. This meant that Ian decided (which was then never being challenged) that he couldn't do **any** homework and felt even worse about himself. A less extreme response by Mum (for example letting Ian be excused from only that homework which he couldn't do after a reasonable try) might have been more helpful here.

Example: Overly high expectations

Mary is the daughter of two high-achieving parents. She's learnt that 'you need to be able to sort things out for yourself in this life'. Actually, Mary is depressed and genuinely can't concentrate. So she simply can't keep up with both her parents and her own expectations. She is often tearful. Her parents insist she still needs to be on the school debating team as 'if she only just tries hard enough she will find she is still just as good at it as she ever was and will feel better'.

Mary thinks of the debate with dread and on the day she can't concentrate well enough to follow what people are saying or put forward her ideas. She takes the arguments of the debate far more personally than they are meant because of her extreme thinking and leaves the debate in tears. A less extreme response from her parents, such as finding something that Mary is presently capable of doing and gradually building things up in agreement with her, would be more helpful here.

Q Have I or have we:

- Been feeling confused about how best to help the young person?

  Yes ☐   No ☐

- Been over-protecting them or wrapping them in cotton wool?

  Yes ☐   No ☐

Q Has this now become unhelpful?

Yes ☐   No ☐

Q Have I or have we been discouraging them from doing anything they find difficult?

Yes ☐   No ☐

Q Has this now become unhelpful?

Yes ☐   No ☐

Q Have I or have we been pushing them harder or faster than is helpful?

Yes ☐   No ☐

Q Has this now become unhelpful?

Yes ☐   No ☐

Write down anything else you have noticed here.

Thinking about the five areas can be a useful way for you and the young person to **together** think about what **is** and what **isn't** helpful at different stages of recovery. For example, helping the young person avoid things they worry about may well help them feel better straight away but can create problems in the long term (because they drop out of daily activities and lose their confidence even more).

Usually it's best to let them move gradually from needing help to taking control themselves again. You (or other key people) may also need to look at your **own** thinking and expectations to see if they have become extreme or unhelpful. (You may find it useful to look at the *Noticing and changing extreme and unhelpful thinking* workbook for ways to do this). You may **yourself** be trying (or expecting someone else) to live up to expectations or to 'rules' that have had their day and are not helpful any more.

Helpful things family and friends can do

The young person may need to make changes in several of the areas and so may need **different** things from you or other people at different stages. The five areas assessment can help you decide, **together**, what is best at any particular time.

The young person may need you for any of these things:

- To recognise and praise their achievements

- To remind them that they matter to you

- For practical help. You can help them by brainstorming practicalities with them, or simply just by not interrupting their attempts to change

- Mainly to support them to gradually return to a fuller, more rewarding lifestyle, even starting with just regular sleep habits

- To keep everything going on around them **as usual** to give them a chance to just have 'normal everyday conversations' that don't focus on their problems

- To be **available** when needed

- Offering an **appropriate** level of support (this may mean 'helping' less)

- Simply to just 'be there' for them, rather than always reassuring them or trying to solve problems on their behalf

- To let them know you do hear and notice even everyday things they say and signals they send out, and that what they say and think actually matters.

You may need to learn to recognise when it's important to let them make changes themselves, rather than letting others take responsibility. You may need to jointly agree with them how and when they may or may not want to share their thoughts and feelings.

When problems have ground people down for a long time, it can be hard to be objective about the present situation or about things in the past. You may be able to offer an important point of view the young person may not currently be aware of. This can help them become more objective and balanced.

The young person may also need you for any of these things:

- To help people listen to each other and think **before** reacting. When there is a problem for someone or a few people in the family, it can be tempting for family members to each withdraw into themselves and focus only on their own problems. Without listening to each other, we can miss the wider picture, especially helpful things that other people in our family could tell us about to help us.

- To let them know you will 'be there' for them for the long term, even if you have disagreements now. You can be a listening ear, encouraging rather than avoiding discussion.

- To encourage them to put into practice what they are learning in this course.

- To keep a positive but realistic outlook that change is possible but will take time. Realising there are no quick fixes.

- To use your sense of humour to cope.

- To plan time for you as well as for others.

- To use coping responses such as relaxation techniques that work well to deal with your own feelings of tension.

- To see a healthcare practitioner for advice if you yourself feel down, depressed or have other health problems.

- To look after yourself and treat yourself well.

- To find out about the problem – through reading (for example this course) and asking healthcare practitioners, to give you the knowledge and skills you need.

You may find it helpful to read a workbook they are working on so you understand the reasons behind what they need to do to make changes. You may also need to look at your own responses to their problem and consider whether any of these are becoming extreme or unhelpful. Perhaps you yourself are overwhelmed by a problem at present or stuck in a situation that is not moving or is left unacknowledged. Do these problems need to be dealt with before the young person can make any changes?

Q Am I doing any helpful behaviours?

Write down what you are doing here.

Q Do I want to develop any of them further?

Write down what you want to try here.

Q Have I got any new ideas to try from this workbook so far?

Write the ideas here.

Staying well and supported ourselves

When we support others we also need to look after ourselves and allow time and space for our own needs. Depression and stress are very common among carers. The danger is that we are so busy offering support that we have no time for ourselves. Sometimes we feel guilty thinking about our own needs, but tackling any distress or upset that you have can often help the young person's emotional problems as well. An adult's own problems or unmet needs can even put pressure on a young person.

Some helpful things you can do for staying well yourself are:

• Having an open discussion of your own stress

• Taking short breaks, weekends or holidays with others

- Plan to have some 'me time' such as having a hobby or going for evening classes or simply relaxing into the day or week

- Attending relaxation or stress management classes or carer support groups

- If necessary, seeing your own doctor to discuss the need for extra treatment and support for the young person. The time you take to do this **is** justified

- Letting yourself accept help from others when it is offered.

Talking about 'it'

It can also be hard to know when and how to talk. When is it best to 'talk about it' and when is it better to keep day-to-day conversation as 'light and cheerful' as possible (meaning serious problems may not be discussed)? There may be place for both, but again extremes in either direction can be unhelpful, and **timing** is important.

Why do we need to communicate?

We need to communicate for many reasons:

- **Praise**. It's important to tell people when they have done something we like or when they have tried hard or done something well. Praise is very powerful and important. People often don't realise that what they have done or even **who they are** has mattered to us. And we often don't say it because we think 'It's too obvious to say' or because of embarrassment. Praise is really important when young people are trying to make positive changes. Letting them know you have noticed (and particularly when you are impressed) is **one of the most powerful things you can do** to keep them motivated, especially as they may well discount their achievements when feeling down. Take **every** chance to do this.

- **Day-to-day communication**. On a daily basis, we all need to communicate simply and clearly to others around us what we need and want. We also need to **hear** what they need and want in return. Where people or families don't do this well, problems can gradually mount up.

- **Clarifying misunderstandings**. Where there is a big difference of opinion or even a 'fight' between people, you will need to acknowledge this openly. Both sides need to be heard for things to move forward or change.

- **Digesting things**. Where someone has had either good or upsetting life experiences, **talking them through with somebody** is a helpful way to digest and understand what they mean for us and to come to terms with them.

*But ... **talking is not the only way to come to terms with things.** People can reflect on life through music, art, sport or other activities. Young people and children, in particular, revisit their experiences again and again 'one step removed' in play as part of normal healthy emotional development. So, people don't have to talk about problems to get over them.*

- **Timing** is important. Sometimes talking about problems or painful issues or thoughts can simply be too painful and too much for us to do **at a particular time**.

- **Whom we talk to about our problems** also plays a part. We often surprise ourselves by being better able to talk to someone we don't know that well than to talk to someone close to us. This is **normal** and **understandable**. Ask yourself: would they be better getting the chance to talk to someone other than me?

- Finally, we **need to listen to and feel heard by each other**. We may need to practise just day-to-day conversation first.

So, ask yourselves:

 Is this a conversation we **need** to have now and is it **possible** now for *us*?

Avoiding communication

All of us are surrounded by people – and have all kinds of friendships and relationships. Our most important relationships are usually with those people whom we live with or with those whom we have lots of contact with – such as immediate family and friends.

When someone we know develops low mood it can be hard to know how best to help. Their distress can affect us too. Sometimes, even just **talking about feeling down** can become a topic that's avoided at home or with friends. This can backfire, because others may be misinformed and misunderstand. And their imaginations may go into overdrive. Here, avoiding talking becomes a problem.

We may even feel embarrassed to discuss things with closer relatives and friends. At times we can avoid this in quite subtle ways, for example steering conversations away from problem areas.

Have I or have we:

● Been avoiding important conversations we need to have?

Yes ☐　　　No ☐

Has this now become unhelpful?

Yes ☐　　　No ☐

● Stopped just spending time together having 'lighter' conversations?

Yes ☐　　　No ☐

Has this now become unhelpful?

Yes ☐　　　No ☐

● Been avoiding talking to others about our problems?

Yes ☐　　　No ☐

Has this now become unhelpful?

Yes ☐　　　No ☐

● Not been really honest with others, for example saying yes when we really mean no?

Yes ☐　　　No ☐

Has this now become unhelpful?

Yes ☐　　　No ☐

● Been avoiding answering the phone or the door when people visit?

Yes ☐　　　No ☐

Has this now become unhelpful?

Yes ☐　　　No ☐

- Been avoiding people or isolating ourselves from friends?

  Yes ☐   No ☐

Has this now become unhelpful?

  Yes ☐   No ☐

- Been avoiding being assertive?

  Yes ☐   No ☐

Has this now become unhelpful?

  Yes ☐   No ☐

- Been completely avoiding asking the person about their problem?

  Yes ☐   No ☐

Has this now become unhelpful?

  Yes ☐   No ☐

Write down anything else you have been avoiding here and if this has caused problems.

Example: Avoiding communication

Ian is 15 years old and has low mood. He lives with his mother, Anne, who has been very supportive and has taken on the role of (overly) protecting him for over a year, excusing him from meeting friends and, often, from attending school.

Anne is now beginning to struggle and is feeling angry at Ian. He has changed so much from the boy she once knew. He sits in his chair watching TV and hardly goes out at all. She is becoming embarrassed whenever friends ask how he is. She is also ashamed about how angry she feels towards him at times.

As a result, Anne is spending more and more time out of the house. She has become active in various local groups, and when she is at home, she tends to spend more time alone in the kitchen or the garden. Anne and Ian rarely talk and so never remind themselves they care for each other and are drifting apart.

The vicious circle of avoidance: Anne and Ian's vicious circle

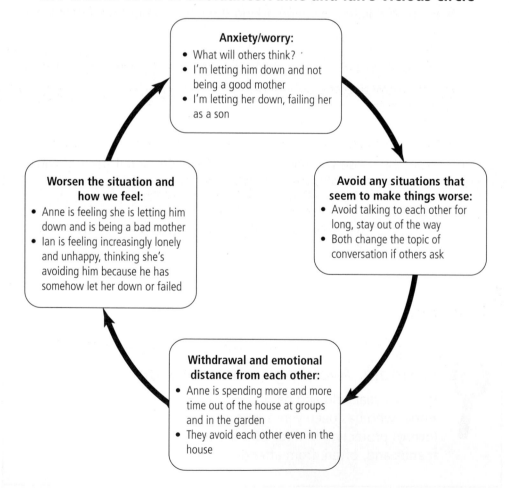

Anxiety/worry:
- What will others think?
- I'm letting him down and not being a good mother
- I'm letting her down, failing her as a son

Avoid any situations that seem to make things worse:
- Avoid talking to each other for long, stay out of the way
- Both change the topic of conversation if others ask

Withdrawal and emotional distance from each other:
- Anne is spending more and more time out of the house at groups and in the garden
- They avoid each other even in the house

Worsen the situation and how we feel:
- Anne is feeling she is letting him down and is being a bad mother
- Ian is feeling increasingly lonely and unhappy, thinking she's avoiding him because he has somehow let her down or failed

Facing the situation together

 Ask yourself (or yourselves):

- Do we **listen** to what the other person has actually said?

- Do we have a way to check if we have understood what they are actually trying to describe?

- Are we **assuming** they want us to 'do something about' or 'give an answer to' the problem, when actually they just need a sounding board to work out what they actually think themselves?

- Have we tended to rush in and jump straight in at the deep end trying to talk about 'the major issue' before we've done these things?

- Did it just end up feeling like a confrontation when we really hadn't meant it to be?

- Do we need to accept that they just do not want to discuss it **now** or **with us**?

Different people will **always** have different experiences of a situation. It's not that some are 'right or wrong' or that anyone is 'lying'.

- Do we actually need to sit down as a whole family to hear where everyone is coming from to discover everyone's experience of the situation – both negative and positive?

- Has the person recovered enough yet to start to see positive things when they talk about the problem, or does talking still lead to a downwards spiral?

Key point

People inevitably often have different opinions about what has happened or should be done. This is a fact of life.

Q How do we as a family deal with times when we have different opinions about something we are upset about or that really matters?

Q Do people feel blamed or criticised or simply pushed aside or ignored?

Q Are we able together to find a way to move forward when people have differences of opinion?

Q We can still love and respect others even when they hold different opinions. Are we able to start to work out what we think together by at least being able to say how different options make us feel, even if we have not worked out yet why we feel that way?

Q Having answered these questions, do we:

• Set time aside to simply be together?

Yes ☐   No ☐

• Actually **listen** to what each other has said?

Yes ☐   No ☐

- Have a way to check/tell each other if we have understood?

  Yes ☐   No ☐

- Try to sort out problems when listening is what is required?

  Yes ☐   No ☐

- As parents or carers show that what the person says is heard and matters?

  Yes ☐   No ☐

- Push too hard or too early to talk about 'the major issue'?

  Yes ☐   No ☐

- Need to discuss this as a whole family to get the whole story?

  Yes ☐   No ☐

- Push the person to talk when they still just get bogged down?

  Yes ☐   No ☐

- Accept and welcome differences of opinion?

  Yes ☐   No ☐

- Share both positive and negative experiences and views?

  Yes ☐   No ☐

- Have a way to move forward together when people disagree?

  Yes ☐   No ☐

Write down anything else you have noticed here.

Key point

Clear communication and children: Children and young people may have all sorts of unrealistic fears if they are kept in the dark. They often worry that they have caused the problem.

Building clear communication

The only way of overcoming communication problems is openness and honesty. Without this, many problems can arise. If you are a person who worries about hurting other peoples' feelings, or aren't quite sure how to discuss these things openly, please read the *Being assertive* workbook.

Remember:

● Make changes slowly – they are more likely to last.

● Choose to spend more positive time together. Go out together if you can.

● Talk to each other – and **listen** even if this is hard to do. Also respect other people's right **not** to communicate.

● Find common ground even if you feel you have drifted apart.

● Make a joint decision about the level of information to give others about the problem. For example, deciding together on a simple one-line reply 'things are much the same or going well' might be enough for most situations.

Here are some things you can say and helpful ways in which you can relate to each other.

● 'This is obviously not a good time to talk, but let's make sure we talk about it later.'

● Sometimes people need to work through an issue by talking at length. Let them talk. Often no comment is needed. Listen for the main message, and then pick up on this point so the person knows you are really listening. For example, 'It sounds like you feel frustrated today because ...'

● Make time to simply enjoy being together.

● Offer praise and encouragement to build confidence. For example, 'I can see such a difference from a month or so ago ...'

- Actively look for things you can comment positively about.

- Try to find at least three positive things to say every day.

Things that don't usually help

Sometimes, friends or family can act in ways that directly worsen the situation for a young person. For example, raising our voice in frustration can make us feel a lot better to begin with but can also have a damaging effect on our relationship and leave us feeling guilty. Similarly, speaking for (or over) the person in social settings can undermine their confidence and make it less likely that they will feel able to tackle their problems.

There can be many reasons for behaving in this way. Often we do these behaviours with good intentions, for example due to concern, friendship and love. Sometimes we do them out of anxiety or, occasionally, even guilt.

Some other examples of unhelpful behaviour are:

- Always talking over or ignoring their day-to-day comments and opinions, especially if they are telling you their needs and you are their parent or carer.

- Offering 'helpful advice' all the time when it isn't appropriate.

- A desire to do **everything** for the person.

- Constantly offering reassurance that everything will work out fine.

- Overly protecting and stifling the person by taking away all their responsibility (and all their choices too).

- Drinking too much or misusing drugs ourselves.

Frustration and anger at helping professionals or even the young person themselves

When someone takes on a supportive or carer role, it's very common to struggle. We can feel demoralised, worried, guilty, frustrated or even angry. These frustrations can spill over into how we talk about helping professionals, for example teachers, social services or healthcare professionals. It can be tempting to become critical and intolerant. But this can undermine a young person's trust in those people. Most professionals can provide helpful support to people. We may have misunderstood what they are trying (or can reasonably be expected) to do. We can also have unsuitable expectations of the young person and feel angry with them.

Wrapping the person in cotton wool

Offering 'extra special attention and support' can also become unhelpful – even if we're doing things with the very best intentions. The relationship may feel **suffocating and frustrating**. The young person can end up feeling like they are much younger and less able than they are. Arguments and little irritations build up and are upsetting for all. Although we mean well, our actions can actually **undermine things**.

When trying to help a person with low mood it's important to encourage them to keep as reasonably active as possible. If we take responsibility for doing everything, the danger is that the person will not be as active as they could be and we create unnecessary dependency. Our good intentions could actually sap the person's confidence.

Similarly, if we allow the young person to dominate us and run their life completely as they wish, their lifestyle may fail completely to meet their social and emotional needs. So they find it hard to have balance between 'give and take' in their relationships. This can then cause a great deal of harm both to them and to their family and wider relationships.

Example: Becoming overly protective

- Mark has reduced activity and is worried by how tired his mother looks. She has banned him from doing any of the housework – even though she is struggling to cope. They are paying a cleaner – and whenever Ian sees her he feels deep shame that he can't do even this. His mum's well-meaning and overly protective actions have undermined how he feels.

- Jane's friends at school have taken over doing her homework on her behalf, and as a result Jane can manage to avoid getting into trouble. While this seems helpful in the short term, in the longer term it prevents her from rebuilding her confidence and has an unhelpful effect on her life.

- Ian's mum often declines invitations for meals out and other social events on his behalf without checking with him first. She doesn't want him to feel pressurised by social events. He is now finding his social life becoming more and more restricted. So he's even more likely to try to go out when he's not feeling up to it if he's asked directly because his feeling is that he's hardly ever asked out any more. His mum does this with good intentions, but it's backfiring in precisely the way she wanted to avoid.

Unhelpful behaviours I may have been doing

Look at the following list and tick any activity you have found yourself doing over the past month. Several **unhelpful behaviours** have been given here to help you to think about the changes that are happening in your own situation.

As a friend or family member, am I or are we:	Tick here if you have noticed this – even if just sometimes
Tending to ignore or not hear everyday things they say, especially if I am or we are their parent(s) or carer(s)	☐
Becoming overly protective of the person – wrapping them in cotton wool	☐
Taking over all responsibility from the person (for example making all the key decisions with no discussion). The result is undermined confidence and often resentment	☐
Having a go at the person from time to time – through frustration or anger	☐
Trying to control **every** aspect of their life	☐
Letting them dominate and have everything as they demand	☐
Talking **only** about how hard things are so that they feel even worse	☐
Advising the person not to try approaches such as this one because of fears that it may do harm	☐
Criticising helping professionals, because they havent been able to find a cure	☐
Undermining or criticising advice that the person has received from a professional	☐
Helping the person avoid doing things because of fears about what harm might result (for example taking over going to shops)	☐
Constantly reassuring the person	☐
Constantly asking about the problem and drawing attention to it	☐
Introducing the person as X, who has this problem, rather than just by their name – you have started seeing the problem rather than a person	☐
Telling the person to avoid any physical activity or exercise as a result of concerns about their mental health	☐

As a friend or family member, am I or are we:	Tick here if you have noticed this – even if just sometimes
Speaking for or over the person in social settings, or in health interviews, etc. You rather than they tell their story	☐
Becoming so focused on the distressed person that other people's needs are not met, for example their brothers, sisters or your partner	☐
Depending on the person to be well and functioning so that they are not 'allowed' to be depressed	☐
Ignoring or avoiding dealing with other very real tensions in the family (for example major problems between parents that is not being acknowledged or dealt with)	☐
Not making time to listen	☐
Not dealing with my or our own problems so that we can't support the young person or be available enough	☐

Making effective changes

Think about how you can begin to make positive changes. This may be:

- **To build up helpful behaviour(s)** – any ideas from doing the checklists above?

- **To reduce unhelpful behaviour(s)** – have you found any you wish to change?

To successfully increase helpful behaviours or reduce unhelpful backfiring behaviours, you need to have a clear plan. Consider ideas that have come to you during your reading of this workbook.

Do

- Plan to alter only **one** key behaviour over the next week.

- Make a **plan** to slowly alter what you do in a step-by-step way, one step at a time and at a pace that is right for the young person until you reach your eventual final goal. Write down your plan in detail so that you can put it into practice.

- Ask yourself the **questions for effective change** (see the *Practical problem solving* workbook) to check that each change is well planned.

- Check **with the young person** whether changes you make are actually helping.

- Make helpful behaviours a regular habit.

Don't

- Choose something that is too ambitious a target to start with.

- Try to start to alter too many things all at once.

- Give in to negative thinking ('nothing can be done, what's the point, it's a waste of time'). Instead, test out if this thinking really is accurate or helpful.

- Make changes without checking with the young person

Faith and seeking help

Sometimes parents or other carers have a strong spiritual belief. This may be very helpful, but sometimes these beliefs can emphasise prayer as the only way towards recovery and healing. We tend to ignore that health workers may play an important part of the recovery process, and they may be part of an answer to prayer. In the same way as you would seek medical help if a child fell from a tree and broke their arm or leg, you need to think about medical help for low mood and depression. If you have doubts about how medical help can help low mood and depression, please discuss this with a spiritual leader whom you respect.

When extra help is needed

These workbooks aim to help young people and their families and friends to make changes themselves. But sometimes a young person may need to be seen by a professional to decide whether other treatments are necessary. We recommend that ideally a person using these workbooks has someone to support them in doing it. But there are times when this will not be enough.

You should get extra help for the young person you're supporting if they have:

- **Severe depression**, for example continuing low mood, tearfulness, significant sleep, concentration, weight or energy loss despite attempts to improve things

- Strong urges to **self-harm** or feeling really **hopeless or suicidal** about the future

- Other concerning **dangerous behaviours**, for example risk-taking, threats of harm to others

- A possibility of immediate or longer-term significant harm or injury by someone else – that is, **physical, emotional or sexual abuse or neglect**

- **Severely withdrawn from life activities**, for example they are missing a lot of school

- **Lost a lot of weight** or are **dehydrated** (their body doesn't have enough fluids to function properly) and they are still refusing food.

There are other situations where extra help is needed or can be a real help. If you or the young person are still worried that something else needs to be done, then it is important to ask for help at least in deciding whether more help is needed.

Sometimes, if a young person is at risk of immediate significant harm (abuse or self-harm), action will need to be taken immediately. There are also professional and voluntary services that can give a great deal of support in the longer term (see details in the next section).

It is always best to get the young person's agreement for getting extra help, but sometimes the risks involved may mean help is needed whether they agree or not. If you are seriously worried that extra help is needed but the young person is refusing, it's still best to ask for help to decide if anything else should or can be done. Don't just keep it to yourself when you should be getting more advice. If you are not sure, you can phone someone fron the list below or NHS Direct (England and Wales) or NHS 24 (Scotland) (see contact details at the end of this workbook) anonymously. These services will help you discuss the issues in confidence and to receive sensible advice as to what to do.

Key point

If you are still worried or concerned, it is better to ask for help or advice than do nothing.

Sources of extra help

- **Family doctor or GP**. The young person's GP can offer medical advice and (if they feel it is necessary) refer them to the Child and Adolescent Mental Health Services (CAMHS) for a detailed assessment.

- **Social services**. Social services can be a great source of support for young people and families with particular needs and problems. You can find your local social services office hours' enquiry phone number and a 24-hour emergency phone number in the *Yellow Pages*.

- The young person's school teacher, head of year, education welfare officer or learning mentor will be best placed to help with school-based problems.

Other organisations you can approach are:

- **ChildLine** (Tel: 0800 1111). This is helpful for children and young people needing advice or just wanting to talk things over. Calls are free and confidential. You can get more information at the ChildLine website (**www.childline.org.uk**).

- **NSPCC**. Adults who are worried about a child can call 0808 800 5000 or visit the NSPCC website (**www.nspcc.org.uk**). Another useful website is www.there4me.com, which is an NSPCC on-line confidential advice resource for children and young people aged 12 to 16 years who are worried about things such as abuse, bullying, exams, drugs and self-harm. The NSPCC has 24-hour helplines (for example NSPCC Child Protection Helpline) that you can call to talk things over without the number appearing on house phone bills.

- Local counselling services, such as **Relate** (see **www.relate.org.uk**).

- **Young Minds** provides information and advice for young people with emotional problems, their families and friends (see **www.youngminds. org.uk**).

- The **Royal College of Psychiatrists** has fact sheets for family and teachers about common mental health problems in children and young persons (see **www.rcpsych.ac.uk**).

- The **Child Psychotherapy Trust** has produced fact sheets about common problems faced by children and young person (see **www.childpsycho therapytrust.org.uk**).

- **NHS Direct** – tel: 0845 4647, 24 hours line; website: **www.nhsdirect. nhs.uk**; or NHS 24 – tel: 08454 242424; website: **www.nhs24.nhs.com**.

You can buy the following helpful books from local or on-line bookshops, or you may find them at your local library. These resources are also available from the bookshop at **www.fiveareas.com**.

- *Overcoming Anxiety: A Five Areas Approach* by Chris Williams

- *Think Good – Feel Good: A Cognitive Behaviour Therapy Workbook for Children and Young People* by Paul Stallard

- *Manage Your Mind: The Mental Fitness Guide* by Gillian Butler and Tony Hope

- *Overcoming Depression and Low Mood: A Five Areas Approach* by Chris Williams

- *I'm Not Supposed to Feel Like This: A Christian Self-help Approach to Depression and Anxiety* by Chris Williams, Paul Richards and Ingrid Whitton

- *Overcoming Low Self-Esteem: A Self-Help Guide to Using Cognitive Behavioural Techniques* by Melanie Fennell

- *Mind over Mood* by Christine Padesky and Dennis Greenberger

- *Young People and Depression Training Pack* by the Depression Alliance

- *Overcoming Your Child's Fears and Worries* by Cathy Creswell and Lucy Willetts

 www.livinglifetothefull.com

This is a free on-line training course that teaches key life skills by using the same model used in this book. It includes useful additional handouts as well as DVD-based videos to learn key life skills confidentially and for free.

Summary

This workbook has covered:

- What happens when a young person has low mood or depression

- What this course is about – and how the young person is using it

- How you can identify helpful and unhelpful responses

- Ways to offer effective support and communicate effectively

- How to look after ourselves and stay well

- How to know when extra help is needed and where to go for it.

My notes